The Weight Loss Habit

The No BS, No Gimmick, (Sort of) Easy Way to Lose Weight and Keep it Off Forever

STEVEN RAY MARKS

ISBN: 979-8-6436-0973-5

CONTENTS

INTRODUCTION: WHY DIETS FAIL

This book isn't going to give you the best health advice.

If your goal is to appear on the cover of fitness magazines or win bodybuilding competitions, stop reading right now. This book isn't for you. There are probably some books that can help you with that, but I have no idea what they are, because I've never had any interest in appearing on fitness magazines.

On the other hand, if you are someone who is overweight, and your goal is to stop being overweight, this is the right book for you. Because unlike other diet books, I'm not trying to give you the *best* advice. I'm giving you *advice you'll actually be able to follow.*

So, you won't be Ms. or Mr. Universe anytime soon. On the other hand, you'll have to buy a whole new wardrobe to replace the clothes that will soon be too big for you. If that's what you want, keep reading.

Most weight loss books are useless. In fact, they're worse than useless.

There are three kinds of weight loss books/plans/diets that don't work.

First, there are the gimmick diets. Like Keto, Atkins, South Beach, Shangri-La, cleanses, boot camps, etc. These can work in the short term. If you want to fit into a wedding dress or show up your old classmates at a high school reunion by pretending to be skinnier than you actually are, these can help you achieve that. But if your goal is to be healthy, these are terrible ideas.

The problem is that these only work for as long as you stay on them. Are you going to give up carbs or have an obnoxious dude dressed up as a drill-instructor scream at you every morning for the rest of your life? Probably not. As soon as you go off these diets, you'll go right back to your old weight. Probably even a higher weight, because you've picked up bad habits from being able to eat as much as you want while on the gimmick diet.

Then you're going through the dreaded weight yo-yo, where you keep losing weight and gaining it back again. This is even less healthy than staying consistently overweight.

The second type are the diets designed by people who Just Don't Get It. These are people who love to exercise, and love to eat healthy. Who live, breathe, and sleep nutrition. Who seem to have infinite time to prepare healthy meals, infinite willpower to resist temptations, and a much faster metabolism than those of us who struggle with our weight. Who think it's fun to hit the gym every day, and that kale tastes better than ice cream. The kinds of people who say obnoxious stuff like "Nothing tastes as good as thin feels."

They put out books saying that to lose weight, all we have to do is eat healthy and exercise more, like we're complete idiots who've never thought of that before. They don't understand the Struggle, because it all comes easy to them.

If you're reading this book, you know the Struggle. How we desperately want to be thinner. The sacrifices we make, forcing ourselves to give up the food we love, and to do exercises we hate, only to fail over and over again. The health nuts have zero clue what that's like.

If you want to learn how to do something that's hard for you, don't ask an expert to whom it comes naturally. Ask someone who faced the same challenges you did, and figured out how to overcome them.

Finally, there are books from people who do know the Struggle, then had some sort of revelation that changed their entire life. Maybe they suffered a heart attack. Or they decided they wanted to be around to walk their daughter down the aisle. Or the clouds parted, and Jesus, Buddha, and Richard Simmons came down from the mountain to tell them they needed to change. And suddenly they went from sitting on the couch eating deep-fried nachos dipped in lard to running fifteen miles a day and eating nothing but steamed broccoli. Then they write a book about how you can do the same.

But realistically, you're not going to change everything about yourself. You're not going to limit your diet to nothing but celery. Because you're a normal person living your life, not someone who had some sort of divine revelation.

At worst, these books put you on the weight yo-yo. At best, they leave you feeling bad about yourself, convincing you that you're a loser and it's your fault you're fat because you couldn't follow their advice.

But it's not your fault. It's the books' fault. They were setting you up to fail. The dirty little secret of the weight loss industry is:

Weight loss books, plans, and diets are written by and for people who don't need them.

This is the reason why some estimates say that up to 95% of people who lose weight through a diet end up gaining it back again. And that's only counting the people who were able to lose weight in the first place.

I beat those odds.

I grew up fat. I made many failed attempts to lose weight. And there were several times where I'd lose a little bit of weight, only to gain it back with interest. I know the Struggle.

And then I hit upon the *right* way to lose weight. Over eight months in 2001 and 2002, I lost 60 pounds. And I've kept the weight off since then. It's not like I'm an underwear model, but I'm at a reasonable and healthy weight. When I tell people I used to be fat, they often don't believe me, because I don't look like it.

This didn't require any sort of divine revelation, or radical change to my life. I didn't have to suffer or go through deprivations. It didn't happen with a snap of my fingers, but it also wasn't terribly difficult. It's probably less challenging than some of the diets you've already tried and failed at. In fact, that lack of challenge is a big part of why it works.

I'm not claiming to be a genius. Honestly, it was mostly blind luck that the tactics I stumbled onto were the ones that worked. It was only years later, when I started reading about psychology and the science of habit-formation, that I really understood *why* they worked.

But the important thing is that they do work.

What exactly are these tactics?

Keep reading.

PROLOGUE: HOW A COMEDY SKETCH CHANGED MY LIFE

If you're wondering who I am to give advice, this tells you my story. If you don't care, and just want to get to the weight loss advice, feel free to skip to Part One. I won't be offended.

It all started with a comedy sketch.

Let me take a step back.

I was always a chubby kid. I'd get my clothes from what was politely called the "husky" section. I was cursed with a slow metabolism, and learned terrible eating habits from my father, who was the kind of guy who would order his corned beef with extra fat, and go back to the buffet for thirds and fourths. (And then needed quadruple-bypass surgery when he was fifty, and died from heart-failure when he was fifty-seven.)

My family tried to spare my feelings by calling this "baby fat" and complimenting me on my broad shoulders, even though I would have been better served by them teaching me proper eating habits and refusing to stock cookies in the pantry.

Then when I hit fourth grade, I became the target for a bully, at the same time that I started suffering from clinical depression. This was before depression was being diagnosed in children. I wouldn't understand what was happening and get properly medicated until I was an adult. I just knew that sometimes I would mentally disappear into a fog. Without the treatment I needed, I self-medicated with food. And that made me balloon up even more.

Even after I escaped the bully that was tormenting me by graduating to a different school, I couldn't escape the depression. I was still a socially awkward weirdo, and being fat certainly didn't make me any more popular.

Eventually I managed to find a group of nerds and outcasts to be my tribe. But by then, my eating habits were set. We'd stay up late into the night playing

Dungeons and Dragons, which is a game where you spend ten hours straight sitting at a table while consuming an entire large pizza, tube of Oreos, and a two liter bottle of Mountain Dew. Or at least, that's how I played it.

In college, I'd hang out for hours in the cafeteria with my friends. We even called ourselves the "Cafeteria Gnomes." And while I was there, why not take advantage of the unlimited food? Grab a snack, another ten chicken fingers, refill my sugary soda, and hit the build-your-own-milkshake bar?

There were plenty of times throughout this period that I *tried* to lose weight. Of course I didn't *want* to be fat. But my diets inevitably failed as I couldn't stick to them. You know, the same thing that happens with everyone who Struggles to lose weight.

By the time I was 23, I was fatter than ever before, had no lovelife to speak of, and, as this was not too long after the dot-com crash, was also unemployed. I was spending my days sitting around watching TV, killing time, and snacking.

I'm giving you this background so you'll know I understand the Struggle. And so you won't scream and throw the book out the window when I tell you the next bit. Because I warn you it's going to sound dumb and obnoxious at first. But please stick with me long enough for me to explain.

The comedy sketch.

I was watching an episode of *The Man Show*, Jimmy Kimmel and Adam Corolla's comedy vehicle before they got super famous. They had a sketch about a new miracle diet called the "Stop Eating So Much" diet.

Of course this sketch was unsympathetic and oversimplifying. It was obviously written by someone who has never had to Struggle with weight, who Doesn't Get it. It failed to understand that people who try to lose weight have far more willpower than those who are naturally skinny. Some might even call it downright cruel.

But despite all that, this sketch would change my life. It would completely alter my relationship to food. Divert my path from following my father to an early grave. And ultimately, shift my entire perspective on the world, not just in terms of diet and health, but for everything.

If you're screaming in rage at this point, I get it. Last chapter I mocked the diet books that tell you all you have to do is eat less and exercise more, as if we've never thought of that.

But after watching this sketch, I thought, "Why not?" Instead of trying a diet based on deprivation, cutting out all the foods I loved, and trying to eat healthy, I decided to try just eating the foods I would normally eat, but less of them. It was just basic math and biology - All else equal, if I was consuming fewer calories, I would lose weight. Period.

Okay, you're probably still furious, because it still sounds like I'm treating you like an idiot. This is all obvious. Consume fewer calories and you'll lose weight. Duh.

It's the *way* I went about doing this. The *strategy* I put in place for ensuring I would consume fewer calories. That was the magic, the secret sauce, the one piece that is missing from all the other diets and why those diets fail.

Anyone can tell you to eat less. Anyone can decide to consume fewer calories. The hard part is figuring out how to do that, and stick to it. Not just today, not just tomorrow, not just over the next three months, but *for the rest of your life.*

Does that phrase *"for the rest of your life"* fill you with sadness or dread? That's why most diets fail.

By the time you finish this book, it won't.

So what is this magic strategy I've been hyping? Well, it's not just one strategy, but many. Which is why this is a book and not a paragraph. However, there's one fundamental idea that all the others stem from. Read on to find out what that is.

STEVEN RAY MARKS

PART I
THE PHILOSOPHY OF WEIGHT LOSS

THE FUNDAMENTAL RULE OF WEIGHT LOSS

Weight loss is all about habits. So is weight gain. In fact, your entire relationship with food is determined by your habits.

To lose weight, you need to change your eating habits.

You may argue that this is an obvious statement, and just kicking the can down the road. How do you change your eating habits?

That isn't necessarily obvious, but at least you're asking the right question.

One of my favorite books is *The Power of Habit* by Charles Duhigg. This talks about the idea of *Keystone Habits*. Frequently, someone looking to change their life will pick up a new good habit or break a bad habit. And this will inspire them to make huge changes throughout their life. For example, someone will quit smoking, and six months later they've lost 50 pounds, are running a marathon, started a business, written a novel, and have a much better relationship with their spouse.

Quitting smoking didn't cause these things. Rather, the keystone habit demonstrates the impact that habit change can have on their life, which leads them to adopt habit change to empower themselves in other areas.

As Duhigg says,

> *"If you believe you can change - if you make it a habit - the change becomes real. This is the real power of habit: The insight that your habits are what you choose them to be. Once that choice occurs - and becomes automatic - it's not only real, it starts to seem inevitable."*

This doesn't answer the question of how to change your habits. And that's because habit change is generally hard. Moreover, to be successful, a habit change needs to be sustainable, which means it's something you're willing to do for the rest of your life.

So what makes a habit change feasible and sustainable? Well, it certainly helps if it's convenient, easy, small, enjoyable, takes minimal time-commitment, offers immediate positive feedback, or is a series of small progressive changes that steadily build up over time.

Giving up the foods you love sucks. Going to the gym four times a week is unpleasant and takes up too much time. That's why you can't keep those habits. (Some people love going to the gym and hate ice cream, so it's easy for them to keep those habits, but if you're reading this book, that probably isn't you.)

The trick is to find the keystone habit, and make it a habit that you will be able to form and keep. Something that's convenient, easy, takes minimal time commitment, offers immediate positive feedback, and will have a big impact on your life.

So what is the keystone habit? The trick that will change your life and make weight loss (sort of) easy?

The fundamental rule of weight loss is to build a lifelong habit of thinking before you eat, make, or buy food, making a rational decision about what and how much to eat, and then to celebrate and take pride in your good decisions.

I'll go into much more depth on this in later chapters, but let me unpack this a bit.

When you are about to purchase food at the store or restaurant, make food, or eat food, take a few seconds to think about it. Note how many calories are in it. Ask yourself whether the enjoyment you get from it is worth the calories. Maybe it is, and that's totally fine. Or is there a diet version or something else you could have that is almost as good, that would be a small drop in enjoyment for a large decrease in calories, and you'd be better off with that? Then think about how much you want to eat. Would you get as much enjoyment from the small size as the large? Could you serve yourself less?

Then comes the easiest, but also the most important part: Anytime you make a wise decision for your health, choosing a lower calorie option or smaller portion than what's available, **take pride in that decision.** Celebrate that you are taking control of your life and your health. Be smug. You are succeeding where so many others fail. You deserve to be proud.

This part is extremely important. Do not skip it. This diet will not work if you are not proud of yourself for being on it.

That last bit may seem a bit wacky. What does pride have to do with food and your metabolism?

To explain, let me take a brief foray into the science of habit formation. (This is explained more in Duhigg's book.)

A habit is where repeated actions form neural pathways in your brain that allow your mind to go into autopilot. Once these neural pathways are formed, it's very easy to slip into them, and very hard to avoid them. Standard diets fail because they're premised on fighting our deeply ingrained habits.

Pausing for a moment to think before you eat doesn't sound too hard. And it isn't. It's certainly easier than any diet plan you can think of. Now that I've made the suggestion, you'll probably do it at your next meal. But will you remember to do it at the meal after that? And after that? And every time you are eating or buying food for the rest of your life? Relying on memory and willpower isn't effective. Only an automatic habit will work.

The trick that I stumbled on was overwriting an existing habit, which is the best and easiest way to change habits.

Habits have what's called a *habit loop*. They start with a cue - something that triggers the habit. Then a routine - the thing you do. Then a reward - something that makes you feel good afterward.

When you eat unhealthy food, your cue is seeing the food. The routine is eating it. The reward is the delicious taste followed by fat and sugar sending pleasurable chemicals to your brain.

Because these have become automated habits, we eat the food without even thinking. But to successfully lose weight, we need to overwrite the habit. We use the same cue - seeing the food. But substitute in a new routine. Actively thinking about if the food is worth it, and making a rational decision about if we really want to eat it, and if so, how much.

But here's where we run into a problem: Where's the reward? If we eat a smaller portion, we still get the delicious taste, but a much smaller hit of fat and sugar. And if we opt not to eat the unhealthy food at all, we don't even get the taste.

If we don't find a substitute for the reward, the habit won't stick, and the diet will fail like so many others. That's where the pride comes in. Pride feels good. Knowing we are taking control of our own lives sends a dopamine hit to our brain.

If we practice this long enough, then eventually instead of craving nachos, we'll start craving good decisions. That's when the habit is formed, and keeping the diet becomes a whole lot easier.

Note that celebrating good decisions does not mean that you should feel shame or beat yourself up if you decide that an unhealthy food is worth eating. Rationally deciding to eat a high-calorie food based on the enjoyment you'll get out of it is not a *bad* decision. In fact, it's good to do this every so often so you don't feel deprived. Otherwise you won't be able to keep to the diet. Just as if you're generally frugal with your money, you still might decide to take an expensive vacation, and wouldn't consider that a bad decision.

I've mentioned "good decisions" several times in this chapter. But I haven't said exactly which decisions are good. That's what the rest of this book is about. A bunch of habits to build and tactics to use to help you lose weight that all share one very important characteristic: **They are easy**. Which means you can put them into practice right now, and keep them in place for the rest of your life. Without struggle, and without feeling like you're missing out.

But ultimately, these all stem from the habit of thinking before you eat. So start building that habit, and start changing your life.

HABITS VERSUS GOALS

What separates success from failure?

Part of it is genetics. LeBron James is naturally taller, stronger, and more coordinated than me, and this contributes to him being better at basketball than me. Similarly, people who are born with a faster metabolism, who enjoy healthy foods, who get a natural high from exercise, will have an easier time maintaining a healthy weight than those of us who don't.

But there's nothing we can do about that.

Part of it is circumstance. People born with rich parents will have an easier time succeeding in life. So will people who were handed the right connections. Or are lucky enough to live in certain countries. If you're surrounded by family members who eat like garbage disposals, keeping thin will be harder than if all your family members are fitness fanatics.

You can't change the circumstances you were born into, and you can't change the past. (You could theoretically change your circumstances going forward, but usually not without radical alterations to your life.)

Part of it is luck. Sometimes the ball bounces a certain way, you bump into the right person, you make a spur of the moment decision that changes your life in unforeseeable ways. But you can't change your luck, and unless you consider your genetics and circumstances to be a matter of luck, luck tends to balance out over time and doesn't really impact your weight.

One thing that *doesn't* separate success from failure is your goal, or wanting things hard enough. Motivational speakers will point to people who have achieved enormous success and tell you that wanting it really hard was what they all had in common. But this is facile. They also all breathe oxygen and poop in toilets.

Yes, enormously successful people wanted it really hard. But so did all the spectacular failures. Because *everyone* has goals. *Everyone* wants to succeed.

When I succeeded in losing weight and keeping it off, I didn't want it any more than all the previous times when I failed. I didn't want it any more than you, or any of the gajillion other people who would love to lose weight. I'm sure there were tons of people who wanted it a hell of a lot more than I did.

What does separate success from failure, other than the factors you have no control over?

Successful people have the right habits.

They are the ones who don't just *want* to succeed, but are doing things every day that will actively move them toward success. This doesn't necessarily mean they're working the hardest, or are the most motivated, or making the most sacrifices - you can work incredibly hard doing something useless. It means that they have found the most effective habits.

Focus on the right habits, and success will follow. Focus on your goals without the right habits, and those goals will forever be an unattainable dream.

There's another problem with thinking in terms of goals rather than habits: Goals are usually a one-shot binary thing.

Let's say you have a goal of losing fifty pounds. Then you lose forty-five pounds. Losing forty-five pounds should be something to celebrate, but you feel like a loser, because you haven't yet achieved your goal. Instead of being motivated by your success, you're demotivated because you're convinced that you're a failure.

Then you finally do reach that fifty-pound milestone. Hooray! You achieved your goal. Enjoy your moment of glory!

Then what? Well, your diet was a success. So you celebrate by buying yourself a cake. And some ice cream. And a pizza. And binge-watching some of your favorite shows. Since you reached your goal, you don't need to worry about your diet or exercise plan anymore.

Then over the next three months, you gain all the weight back.

With a habit, you'll lose the fifty pounds, and keep it off. And keep going. You won't have the artificial milestone to celebrate, but there will be plenty of natural milestones: When you can climb stairs without getting winded. When you realize you need to buy smaller sized clothes. When you wear a bathing suit without feeling embarrassed. When you tell someone you used to be fat and they don't believe you.

Those are the things that are genuinely worth celebrating - far more than an arbitrary number.

In self-help literature, this idea is often referred to as "Systems vs. Goals," first coined by Scott Adams, the cartoonist behind Dilbert. I prefer to look at it as Habits vs. Goals. *Systems* is broader and more encompassing. *Habits* become automatic and easier over time. That's the more focused approach I'm using in this book.

EASY VERSUS BEST, DIETARY RESTRICTIONS, AND ALTERNATIVE DIETS

Let me tell you a little story about my mother. My mother read the book *Better Than Before* by Gretchen Rubin. (Which is an excellent book. I'm a big fan of Gretchen Rubin's work and her *Happier* podcast.) In this book, Rubin mentioned that she had stopped eating carbs, and it made her generally feel better.

After reading that, my mother decided that she was also going to give up carbs. Completely. For the rest of her life. And then she followed through on it. She hasn't eaten any carbs since.

She's willing to do things like order avocado toast without the toast. And she lost thirty pounds in a matter of months.

If you're the kind of person who can do that, great! But if that describes you, you're probably already skinny and you aren't reading this book. (Unless you actually are my mother, reading this book because her son wrote it, in which case, "Hi Mom. Love you.")

But what about the rest of us?

I started this book by saying I wasn't going to give you the best health advice.

Why don't I want to give you the best health advice? Because the *best* health advice is complicated, hard, time-consuming, and unpleasant. The *best* thing for your health would be to spend three hours a day making freshly prepared perfectly balanced healthy low-calorie meals, carefully checking all of the nutrients against elaborate tables, checking the component amino acids against their hormone cycles, and whatever else is the latest fad coming out of Shape Magazine.

But who wants to do that? Not you. Which is why you don't do it.

Pretty good advice you actually follow is infinitely better than great advice that is so mind-bogglingly complicated that it makes your head spin and convinces you to eat an entire pizza instead.

Maybe giving up carbs entirely is the best health advice. I think the science is still out on that, but it could be true. But regardless of its effectiveness, it isn't something most people can do for their entire lives.

That's why I stick to pretty good advice that is easy.

I'll say a lot of things in this book that will make health nuts gasp and drop their organic kale smoothie. For example, I fully encourage you to eat fast food. I have an entire chapter on how you can eat fast food and lose weight, as long as you do it the right way. And frozen meals are even better - that's one of your best tools.

Another area where I've consciously chosen to keep the diet less than perfect is that I focus almost exclusively on calories.

"But the science of weight loss has progressed beyond simple calories!" People Who Don't Get It might complain. What about carbs, and saturated fats, and Omega 3s, and good calories and bad calories, processed foods, and how sugars cause inflammation, and whatever the latest research that's changing so fast nobody can possibly keep up with it says?

And that's the problem. Nobody can keep straight the constantly changing landscape. If you try, you'll end up so bewildered you won't get around to actually building the habits you need to lose weight.

Are all calories the same? No. Is it close enough that focusing on calories will do a pretty good job of helping you lose weight? Yes. So that's what we do. And then you've just got one number to care about.

What about dietary restrictions? First of all, if your doctor has put you on a certain diet, do what your doctor says. Obviously.

What if you have allergies, or are vegan, or vegetarian, or gluten free, or low carb, or paleo, or intermittently fasting, or locavore - for ethical reasons, or health reasons, or because it makes you feel good, or just because you feel like it? Well, since my diet is more of a philosophy of how you look at food, it's entirely compatible with any other dietary restrictions. So if you want to do any of those, knock yourself out.

WILLPOWER IS LIKE A MUSCLE

Let's say you want to become a weightlifter. (You probably don't *actually* want to become a weightlifter - if you did, you'd be reading strength training books instead of this one. This is just a hypothetical.)

You wouldn't attempt to bench-press a 300-pound barbell on your first day. If you tried, you'd either fail to move it at all, or end up hurting yourself.

You start off lifting the weights that are within your capability. You keep doing those reps, and your muscles grow. As you get stronger, you gradually increase the weight, and over months or years, build up to being able to bench that 300-pound weight.

Willpower is the same way. And this is another reason why traditional diets fail.

Traditional diets ask you to make all of the changes all at once. To adopt a perfectly healthy diet immediately. To sacrifice all the foods you love, and take the time and make the effort to do the exercises you hate, right off the bat. This is the equivalent of lifting the 300-pound weight on your first day.

You haven't built up your willpower muscle yet. When you try to do something beyond your capabilities, you completely fail, and fall back into your old routines. Or worse, you injure your willpower. You say, "Screw this," and collapse onto the couch to binge-watch Real Housewives while eating an entire tub of ice cream.

This is nothing to be ashamed of, any more than you should be ashamed that you can't walk into a gym and lift a 300-pound weight without any training.

This is another way that Keystone Habits work. When you adopt a Keystone Habit, you are exercising your willpower muscle. This is the equivalent of putting in the reps on the lighter weights. You are making your willpower, and yourself, stronger. So that you build up a more powerful willpower muscle that is better able to do the more challenging things.

Then you add another habit to it - you're doing reps with a heavier weight. So you become stronger. And it's easier to add a third habit. And it keeps getting easier and easier.

Now, imagine you're a competitive weightlifter, about to go on stage to demonstrate the maximum you can lift. You'd probably do some warm-ups first. (I assume - I don't actually know much about weightlifting.) But would you work yourself to the point of exhaustion, so your arms feel like jelly right before it's time to do the lift that counts?

Of course not. You know that your muscles can get fatigued.

So can your willpower. The more you use your willpower throughout a day, the less of it you have available. While using willpower strengthens it in the long-term, it weakens it in the short-term.

Which means late at night, after you've dealt with a stressful day at work or school or dealing with kids and crises at home, is when you're likely to make the worst decisions about your health.

It would be nice if we could wave a magic wand to get rid of all the stress and hard stuff we have to deal with throughout the day. But that's not realistic. So we shouldn't form a plan that relies on willpower in the evenings after a hard day. Throw one more reason onto the pile of why traditional diets don't work.

There isn't any way to get around human nature, how willpower works, and how our lives are structured. Instead of making a futile effort to fight it or wish it away, we need to accept it and come up with a plan to achieve our goals based on how the world actually *is* and not on how we would *prefer it to be*. This means putting in the training to build our willpower muscle, developing tactics that reduce the need for willpower, and trying to arrange things such that we make the decisions that require willpower at a time when our willpower is stronger.

How do you actually do that? See the next section of the book for specific strategies.

ACCEPT THAT IT'S UNFAIR

Everyone knows that one person that can eat like a stoned grizzly bear and not gain any weight.

They'll down an entire bucket of KFC and two boxes of Oreos in one sitting, go back for seconds, and still look good in a swimsuit. And you want to punch them in the face.

Then people will tell you that you could look like them if only you had more self-control.

You also know someone who runs ultra-marathons for fun, and the gym is their happy place. They're high on life or endorphins, and don't understand why we won't do a triathlon with them. Because they enjoy exercise, it takes no more willpower for them to work out than it would take for us to plop down on the couch with a bag of Cheetos.

Some people love exercise. And those who do tend not to understand that for the rest of us, exercise is somewhere between boring and painful.

I mentioned earlier that a heavy person likely has far more willpower than a thin person. Because when someone is naturally skinny, it doesn't take any willpower to maintain that. But someone who is heavy is constantly struggling against their own body, exercising their willpower to lose weight, or to not be heavier than they already are.

Naturally skinny people have Thin Privilege, and it's not fair.

But whining about how unfair this is isn't going to take inches off your belly. It isn't going to improve the health of your heart. It isn't going to help you live a better life.

If you want to lose weight, you need to accept that it's unfair you've been cursed with a crap metabolism, bad habits, and counterproductive tastes, and then move on and take ownership over your own diet and weight.

It's not fair. Other people have it easier. But no matter how much you complain, no matter how much you get skinny people to recognize their Thin

Privilege, nobody can lose weight for you but you.

THE CALORIE EQUATIONS AND EQUILIBRIUM WEIGHT

In a previous chapter, I talked about how I boil everything down to calories. It's oversimplifying, but it's good enough. To oversimplify things more, there are two equations you ought to keep in mind:

1.   Calories Burned - Calories Consumed = Weight Lost

If you burn more calories than you consume, you will lose weight. Period, end of story. That is how you lose weight on a fundamental level.

On the other hand, if you consume more calories than you burn, so the equation comes out negative, you will gain weight.

How much weight will you lose or gain? That's the second equation:

2.   3,500 Calories = 1 Pound (Or 7,700 Calories = 1 Kg)

Take the current amount of food you're eating as a baseline. For every 3,500 calories that you cut out from that, you'll lose a pound. This is approximate, it will vary from person to person, and even within an individual over time, but it's a good rule of thumb when evaluating food.

But there's a complication here:

Your body consumes calories just by existing. The heavier you are, the more calories it will consume. Because whenever you walk, you have to haul around more weight. Your heart has to pump a larger amount of blood to more volume of body. When you breathe, you're moving more chest. This means that the more weight you lose, the fewer calories you're naturally burning. So weight loss keeps getting harder.

Eventually you'll reach a point where everything you've been doing to lose weight up until then is just keeping you at the current weight, and you don't lose any more. This is what I call your equilibrium weight.

Your equilibrium weight is a function of the amount of daily activity you get, your daily caloric input, and your own individual metabolism. Different people living the same lifestyle and eating the same food will have different equilibrium weights, because they have a different metabolism. And for a single individual, their equilibrium weight will change based on how many calories they regularly consume and how much exercise they get. You don't have to be on a diet to hit an equilibrium weight. You'll have one for any amount of calories and activity.

Equilibrium weight explains another of the many reasons most diets fail. The calorie equations can work for you in the short run, but against you in the long run.

Say you go on a diet. Every day, you consume 1,000 fewer calories than you normally do. After 28 days, you've cut out a total of 28,000 calories, and in keeping with the calorie equations, you've lost eight pounds. (28,000 / 3,500 = 8)

Then you say, "Hooray! I fit into those pants that were too tight! I met my goal." You stop the diet, and go back to your old eating habits.

But now you're eight pounds lighter. Your body isn't burning as much as it used to. Before the diet, you were at your equilibrium weight. Now you're burning fewer calories, but still consuming the pre-diet amount. Your calories consumed is greater than your calories burned, so you start gaining that weight back. And you keep gaining it, until you reach your old equilibrium weight, where the calories burned is back to the same as the calories consumed.

This is the dreaded weight yo-yo.

But wait. It's actually worse than this. Because while you were on your diet, you were training your metabolism to get by on fewer calories. Now it isn't burning as much. Since your metabolism has changed, your equilibrium weight has actually shifted higher, and you'll end up heavier than before you started, even if you have the exact same eating habits.

This is why you need to be careful with the calorie equations. Only use them for permanent changes - habits you'll keep for life. Temporary deprivations will come back to bite you.

FIGURE OUT HOW MANY CALORIES ARE RIGHT FOR YOU

Fundamentally, there are two reasons you might be overweight: You eat more calories than a healthy person, or you have a slower metabolism and need fewer calories than a healthy person. (Or both.)

You will need to figure out which of these is your problem, or if both of them are. Either way, the solution is to consume fewer calories. But if you have a slower metabolism than a healthy person, you will need to consume fewer calories than what is considered normal.

For me, the problem was both. I had unhealthy eating habits. But even if I ate the recommended number of calories, it would have been too much.

I can't tell you how many calories will be right for you, because it will depend on your own metabolism and lifestyle. You'll have to dial in on that. Crash diets can be unhealthy. If you're within 50 pounds of your goal weight, and you're losing more than 1 to 2 pounds a week, you should consider slightly increasing the number of calories you consume.

For me, I realized I was consuming too few calories when I got *too* skinny. My ribs were sticking out and I got dizzy when I stood up quickly. I realized I needed to slightly increase my calories per day. Though I didn't realize I needed to increase my caloric intake until I reached an equilibrium weight that was too low, after eight months of building up various habits that allowed me to steadily drop weight.

It may not be clear to you what the right number of calories are until you level off at an equilibrium weight, so this is something to look out for.

EATING HABITS HAVE A BIGGER IMPACT THAN EXERCISE

I once went to a talk by someone who, like me, had beaten the odds to lose weight and keep it off long-term. I was curious what his strategy was, and how it differed from mine.

His method was quite simple: He got rid of his car, and used his bicycle to get everyone he needed to go. He had a lengthy commute, so this amounted to four hours a day on the bike.

How did he get his kids to school, or buy groceries? I dunno. I guess that was his wife's problem.

You're not going to do that, because that's crazy.

Exercise is great. It has lots of health benefits. You should totally exercise. I have a chapter later on easy(ish) ways to build exercise habits.

But unless you go to crazy extremes like riding a bike four hours a day, exercise by itself is not an effective way to lose weight.

"But wait," you may say if you're the kind of person who likes to argue with books. "What about the calorie equations? If I increase my calories burned, I'll lose weight."

That would be true if all you did was increase calories burned. But when you exercise, you make yourself hungrier. And you make yourself feel like you deserve a treat. So you end up eating more. Weight loss comes from consuming fewer calories than you burn. If you increase *both* your calories consumed and your calories burned, it's not going to help you lose weight.

Often people who embark on an exercise plan without a change to their eating habits end up *gaining* weight, because they'll assume that the exercise gives them license to eat even more. Or worse, they'll reward themselves with some high calorie treat after the exercise.

Additionally, people tend to drastically overestimate just how many calories they burn through exercise. If you spend twenty minutes on a treadmill and then drink a Gatorade, you've probably consumed more calories from the Gatorade than you burned on the treadmill, and left yourself worse off weight-wise.

Now, even if you do increase your calories burned and your calories consumed by the same amount such that you don't lose any weight, this isn't a bad thing. You're still getting all of the other benefits of exercise. And that's great. I fully encourage you to do this.

But if you want to lose weight, you need to focus on your eating habits more than your exercise habits.

DON'T LET A SLIP UP MAKE YOU GIVE UP

Nobody's perfect. We all have bad days. We all have setbacks. And that's okay.

A lot of people have a tendency to fall off a diet, eat a bunch, and then say, "Oh well. I ruined my diet, so I guess that's over."

Don't do that.

If you ate too much yesterday, you can still eat a healthy amount today. And tomorrow, and the day after that.

Remember, eating better is a commitment you are making **for the rest of your life**. That doesn't mean you'll eat healthy *every single meal* for the rest of your life. That's wildly unrealistic.

There will be days that you make the rational decision that it is worthwhile to pig out. And there will be days that you lose your self-control and pig out without meaning to.

That's fine. I do that. Everyone does that. You don't think there are days when Heidi Klum sneaks away from her personal trainers and private chefs to secretly snarf down a pizza?

Don't do it every meal. Don't make a habit of it. Try not to do it every week even. But if you occasionally overindulge, that's perfectly acceptable - even healthy. (From a mental perspective.)

Just go back to eating healthy after that.

BELIEVE YOU CAN BE SKINNY

This is extremely important:

You have to believe you will succeed in your diet, and will eventually be skinny.

I know you've been dealing with The Struggle your whole life. Maybe you've failed at diets dozens of times. Maybe you've been overweight for so long that you see that as part of your identity. And you don't think it will ever change.

Do not think this way!

This diet is different. Remember, I Struggled with weight my whole life, until I found the *right way* to lose it. Now that you are doing it in the right way, you will be able to lose it too. **It is extremely important that you believe this.**

This isn't a Law of Attraction type thing. Regardless of your feelings on the Law of Attraction, this point is unrelated to that.

This is based on your own internal psychology. Just believing that you will be skinny on its own isn't enough to make you skinny. You have to put in the effort to change your habits, and reduce your caloric intake. But belief is a necessary component to this.

Because if you *don't* believe you will succeed, then you will fail. You won't put in the work to build the habits, or you won't maintain them, or you'll give up at the first setback.

You have to believe you can do it. And you **should** believe you can do it. Because you are armed with the secret to building the habits that make weight loss (sort of) easy.

IT EVENTUALLY GETS EASIER

The benefit and the curse of habits is that, well, they're habitual. Okay, that sounds like a silly tautology. But it's true.

The longer and more consistently you keep a habit, the more automatic it becomes. Your brain is forming and strengthening neural pathways so that when you encounter the same stimulus, you will follow the same behavior with no thought or willpower necessary.

You may complain that the Weight Loss Habit is about engaging in conscious thought before you eat, so I'm being contradictory when I say that eventually it will become something that happens without conscious thought. If you brought up that objection, good. You've been paying attention.

That is a paradox. But remember, when you are thinking before you eat, make, or buy food, making a rational decision about what and how much to eat, and then celebrating and taking pride in your good decisions, the ultimate goal is to *make those good decisions*. And **that** is what will become more automatic.

Healthy food and smaller portions will become your default. What you think of "lunch" will be a Lean Cuisine and not an Epic Burrito with extra chips and guac. A "snack" will be an apple instead of a king-sized Snickers.

You'll still be taking a moment to think before you eat. But it will be a very short moment when it's healthy food, which will be most of the time. You'll be taking a longer time to think on the much rarer occasions when you're contemplating eating a larger amount of unhealthy food.

But it goes beyond this. Over time, you'll experience physical changes as your stomach shrinks, and mental changes as you build a new life around your thinner body. After long enough, your actual desires will change. Not necessarily for the kinds of food you eat, but for the amounts. You won't *want* to overeat.

There will come a time when that third trip to the buffet or polishing off the four-course dinner or eating every scrap of the heaping plate of barbecue seems as appealing to you as a big pile of dog poop. It doesn't take any willpower to resist because eating it just seems gross.

I can't tell you how long that will take. It may be six months; it may be ten years. But if you consistently keep up the Weight Loss Habit, it *will* happen eventually.

And that is when you win.

PART II
STRATEGIES TO MAKE WEIGHT LOSS (SORT OF) EASY

PART II INTRODUCTION

In the previous section, I laid out the fundamental rule of weight loss. As a reminder, this is:

The fundamental rule of weight loss is to build a lifelong habit of thinking before you eat, make, or buy food, making a rational decision about what and how much to eat, and then to celebrate and take pride in your good decisions.

But what is a "good" decision? It's not limiting yourself to eating nothing but kale. In fact, that would be a terrible decision. Because that would be creating an impossible standard you're not capable of keeping, which sets you up for failure and ultimately rage-quitting your diet.

A good decision is one that balances keeping you healthy with keeping you happy, and is accomplished through building eating habits that you will be capable of keeping.

The previous section was about the philosophy and theory of how to realistically lose weight and keep it off. This section is about the pragmatic, nuts and bolts, specific techniques you can use.

HOW TO USE THIS SECTION

Every individual is different. We all have different tastes, abilities, strengths, and weaknesses. Certain things are hard for some people and easy for others.

Read through each of the chapters. As you do, think about how easy or difficult the strategy would be for you to implement.

Each of these tactics by themselves should be fairly easy for most people. But we all have our hang-ups. You will probably find a few that you balk at, where you either recognize that they will be hard for you, or you simply don't want to do them. And that's fine.

Whether or not you find any strategies that seem hard to you personally, here is the important thing: **Do not try to fully implement all of the strategies at once.** If you try to do that, you will fail. You simply cannot change twenty different habits at once. That's not how habit formation works. Don't try it.

Find the strategies that seem like they will be the easiest for you to implement. And choose a few of them to start off with. I can't tell you how many, because that's going to depend on just how easy they are for you personally, and on your own willpower muscle and habit formation. But however many you *think* you can handle, do one or two fewer than that.

(You may find that there are some strategies you're already using, or that aren't applicable to you. In that case, you can ignore those.)

Keep practicing those habits you've chosen until you're following them consistently and they become second nature. Once that happens, add a few more habits. When those are second nature, add some more. Keep doing this, adding habits in order of difficulty, easiest to hardest.

While going through this process, frequently look back through this section. Try to occasionally use the strategies from the chapters you haven't yet incorporated into your habits. Not all the time, and don't feel bad about yourself when you don't do this. But it's good to get some practice in before you officially try to incorporate the habit. It will make adopting it much easier. (And you may find that the occasional practice turns into all-the-time, and you end up accidentally adopting the habit without even intending to. If that happens, you should feel extra good about yourself.)

Then when it comes time to tackle the last few habits, the ones that seem the hardest, you'll have built up your willpower muscle, and built the habit of adopting habits. And you'll find them to be far easier than you thought they would be when you started.

But if they're still too hard, or still something you just don't want to do, that's also okay. Making 80% of the good decisions is nothing to scoff at. You might not get down to the same equilibrium weight as if you were making 100% of the good decisions, but you'll be a lot better off than when you began.

So let's get started. Here are the tactics to change your life.

SWITCH TO DIET SODA

Lots of things in life are hard. Then there are some things that are so incredibly easy that you just want to shake people and ask them, "Why the hell aren't you doing this already?"

This is one of the latter things.

If you drink sugary soda, switch to diet soda instead.

Do this. Right now. Never drink sugary soda again.

This takes absolutely zero time, effort, willpower, or cost. Just order a Diet Coke instead of a Coke. That's all you have to do. Every restaurant or store that stocks Coke also stocks Diet Coke. They're right next to each other. They're the same price. You don't have to put in any work, or stop to think, or make any changes to your behavior or lifestyle.

This will make a significant impact on your health in exchange for literally no effort. That's an infinite return on investment.

Let me repeat myself. **Switch to diet soda right now.**

A can of Coke has 150 calories. A can of Diet Coke has zero calories. If you drink two Cokes a day, switching to Diet Coke eliminates 109,500 calories a year. That's 31 pounds that you can lose for free.

Losing 31 pounds won't get you on Oprah, but when you consider you don't have to put in any effort at all to lose it, it's a downright miracle.

Don't like the taste of diet soda? Force yourself to drink it for a few days and you'll get used to it. In fact, after a few weeks you'll likely find that you no longer like the taste of corn syrup, and actively prefer diet soda.

Worried about artificial sweeteners? Maybe if you ate seventeen million pounds of pure aspartame it's possible it could theoretically increase your risk of cancer by a fraction of a percent. But that's nothing compared to the very real health effects of obesity.

You can expand this idea beyond soda. Use artificial sweetener instead of sugar in your coffee. And this may make you Southerners gasp, drop your best deviled egg plate, and say "Bless your heart," but you're allowed to put Splenda in your sweet tea. It's true. My wife is a genuine Southerner, and she does this to make no-calorie tea so sweet it hurts your teeth. Buy the zero calorie Gatorade or Powerade. Ocean Spray makes excellent diet cranberry juice, as well as many flavors of diet cran-[insert other fruit here] juice. Use Splenda instead of sugar when you're baking - you can find baking Splenda at any grocery store.

There's no such thing as a free lunch, but there is a free way to lose weight, and this is it.

Do this now!

LEAVE FOOD ON THE PLATE

Here's a couple pieces of advice you've probably heard a gajillion times:

"When you get your food in a restaurant, immediately get a take-home container, and put half the food into it."

"Stop halfway through your meal, and wait fifteen minutes before continuing, to see if you're still hungry."

These are excellent pieces of advice, and great ways to keep from overeating, except for one thing:

Nobody does them.

Seriously, have you ever done these things? Have you ever even *seen* anyone do either of these things? I haven't.

Ordering a take-home container immediately makes you feel like a weirdo freak. And as for pausing your meal for fifteen minutes, you're probably too distracted by your conversation, or watching TV, or whatever else you're doing while eating to remember to do that. And if you're eating with friends, are you going to make them all wait for you?

Then there are the people who tell you to practice *mindful eating*, as if we aren't busy people living busy lives, and we have time to turn our meal into a meditation session.

Let's start with something simpler.

Most of us have the habit of eating all the food that's set in front of us. If it's on the plate, we finish it. If it's in the McDonalds bag, we eat it. We gobble up the entire slice of cake that's served to us.

But there's no law saying we *have* to do that.

Stopping halfway through is hard. But what about leaving just the last bite? That doesn't sound too hard, does it?

When you leave one bite on the plate, you're still getting to enjoy almost as much delicious food. Your brain and stomach are getting pretty much the same amount of enjoyment. You're just stopping one bite early. So work on building that habit.

The last chapter about switching to diet soda was something incredibly easy that would have a huge impact. By contrast, this won't have an enormous impact directly, and is harder than it sounds.

If you were serving yourself 98% as much food, that would be easy. But once it's on the plate, stopping yourself before that last bite becomes much harder. You've got to snap yourself out of your automatic habit of cleaning the plate. Bring yourself back to the process of eating. Actively, think, instead of just following your habits. That is challenging.

(Don't forget to be proud of yourself every time you succeed at doing this.)

So why do this? What's the value? I mean, realistically that one bite of food isn't going to make a huge difference to your calories consumed or your waistline.

There are a few reasons. First of all, this is an exercise to strengthen your willpower muscle. This little effort you put in at every meal will make it easier for you to resist the big temptations.

Second, you are proving to yourself that you have control over the plate, instead of the plate being your master. You are a rational thinking human with your own agency. Food being on a plate does not mean that you are compelled to eat it. You make your own decisions about what to eat. And by leaving a bite on the plate, you are proving that to yourself. Once you have proven that to yourself, it gives you more control over everything that you eat.

Finally, it doesn't have to be only one bite. Once you have mastered this habit, you'll realize you can leave far more food on the plate. Leave half the food on the plate, or two thirds. Only eat what you actively want to eat. This is how you build up to that ability. And when you are able to do that, then it starts making a real difference to your calories consumed.

One final note about this: You may feel a tinge of guilt about wasting food, especially if you grew up with a parent nagging you to clean your plate because there are kids starting in Africa. Don't think that way. Eating food you don't need is not going to help starving third world children in any way.

USE SMALLER PLATES

It sounds a bit silly, but this is a very simple, no-effort way to lose weight. Just start using smaller plates. You may have to go out and buy some, or else use salad/appetizer dishes instead of entree dishes. Or use a saucer as a plate - I promise I won't tell anyone at charm school about this shocking breach of etiquette.

Humans have a tendency to judge things comparatively. A big plate without a lot of food on it looks *wrong* somehow, so there's a natural inclination to add more food in order to correct the imbalance. When your goal is to consume less food, you want to avoid this. You could try to rely on willpower, or constantly reminding yourself to avoid this pitfall. But remember: We want to make weight loss easy. And it's much easier to just use a smaller plate, so the ratio of food to plate size looks right with a smaller amount of food to begin with.

By contrast, trying to put too *much* food on a small plate will look wrong, and be something that you automatically avoid, meaning the smaller plate will make eating less food your default.

And at a certain point, adding additional food to the small plate will be outright impossible. If you want to eat more, you'll have to make a conscious decision to get a second plate or larger plate to accommodate the additional food. Forcing yourself to make that conscious decision is also forcing yourself to pause and think about if it's worthwhile. Or in other words, to practice the Weight Loss Habit.

A related tip is to use green-colored plates. Most green foods are vegetables that are low in color. They'll blend in with the plate, so you'll instinctively use more of them, filling yourself up while consuming fewer calories. While most high calorie foods are colors that contrast with green, so you'll instinctively put less of them on the plate.

The effect is small, and there are plenty of exceptions. I wouldn't suggest you spend the money to replace perfectly good dishware for this. But if you're buying new dishes anyway, this is a reason to lean toward green ones.

ASK RESTAURANTS TO BRING YOU LESS FOOD

Just because you paid for food doesn't mean you need to eat it. And it doesn't mean you need to take it. Even better than leaving food on your plate is not putting it on your plate in the first place. Then you don't even have the temptation.

When you're ordering at a restaurant, you can tell them "Hold the fries," or "You don't need to bring bread to our table," or "Half the usual amount of mashed potatoes."

It will make it easier for you to not overeat. Plus you can get a warm fuzzy for helping out the environment by not wasting resources. And you're saving your favorite restaurant a little bit of money.

FIND LOW CALORIE SUBSTITUTES FOR HIGHER CALORIE FOODS

I'm not going to lie to you: Diet ranch dressing doesn't taste as good as regular ranch dressing. It just isn't the same thing.

Regular coffee with some sugar-free Torani syrup doesn't taste as good as a caramel macchiato.

Vegetable-based pasta substitute doesn't taste like real pasta. Turkey burgers aren't as good as real hamburgers.

Lean Cuisine frozen pizzas or home-made pizzas with cauliflower crust aren't as good as deep-dish Chicago-style from your favorite pizzeria.

Skim milk doesn't taste as good as whole milk.

And those dairy-free ice cream substitutes made out of god-knows-what do not taste the same as Ben and Jerry's.

But they're reasonably close. Sure, in a taste-test you could easily tell the difference. But the low-calorie substitutes are *good enough*.

You can put low calorie ranch dressing on your salad, and it will still be healthy, while regular ranch dressing makes it just as bad for you as french fries.

You can eat half a pint of ice-cream substitute and it's only 150 calories.

Lean Cuisine frozen pizzas range from 310 to 400 calories. You'd probably end up consuming more like 1500 calories if you eat a few slices of normal pizza. (Cauliflower crust pizzas have a huge range, depending on how they're made, so be sure to check their nutrition info. Some are much healthier than traditional pizzas, and some aren't. At California Pizza Kitchen, there's only 7 calories per slice difference between their regular crust and their cauliflower crust!)

You can use cauliflower rice and vegetable-based pasta instead of regular rice and pasta. Personally, I think these actually taste better than the originals, but even if you disagree, the difference in calories is probably worth the difference in taste.

You can drink light beer for ⅔ the calories of regular beer. Or if you're just drinking to get a buzz on, you can have a shot of hard alcohol mixed with a diet soda. (FYI, a glass of wine has slightly fewer calories than a bottle of beer, but it's not a huge difference.) If you're getting a mixed drink, have vodka mixed with diet cranberry juice instead of a pina colada.

You don't have to sacrifice the foods you love. If you can find lower calorie substitutes that are almost as good, you just have to sacrifice a little bit of quality.

Would you rather eat Ben & Jerry's and be fat, or be skinny and eat something that's 85% as tasty? Seems like an easy choice to me.

MAKE CHANGES WITH OTHERS, OR EAT ON YOUR OWN

I mentioned previously that in many ways, I stumbled into the secrets to weight loss through dumb luck rather than actively figuring them out. There was one aspect that gave me a huge leg up which I never even realized until many years later.

While I was trying to lose weight, I was single. For part of that period, I was unemployed. And when I got a job, it was in a high-demand environment where I didn't have time to go out to eat and would instead eat lunch at my desk.

This was hugely advantageous, because it meant I didn't have a family or coworkers to share meals with. I was planning and eating meals by myself.

Any changes I made to my diet were changes that only impacted me. I didn't have to explain or discuss them with anyone else. I didn't have to observe how others were eating.

People are enormously affected by those they spend time with. If you eat with others, the way they eat is going to influence the way you eat.

If your family members, friends, coworkers, or other people that you regularly eat with are trying to improve their eating habits at the same time you are, that is ideal. You can try to change the same habits at the same time. This will make it easier for all of you to succeed. You can keep each other on track. Eat the same healthy meals. Do the same healthy things.

If your meal-mate(s) eat healthy and you've previously eaten poorly, that is also a good situation. You can announce to them that you are trying to eat better. Or don't, if you're worried that they'll overwhelm you with health-nut advice. Either way, they'll be a positive influence on you.

But what if your meal-mate(s) eat unhealthily and have no interest in changing? Or worse, are blessed with a fast metabolism while you're cursed with a slow one, so it's perfectly healthy for them to eat far more food than you should.

This is going to make it much harder for you. Being around people who eat more calories than is healthy for you makes it much more likely that you will fail in your efforts to lose weight and keep it off. Sorry, but that's the reality.

So how do you handle this, short of leaving your family, quitting your job, or accepting that you'll forever be fat?

You're going to have to explain to your family, co-workers, or other meal-mates that you'll be eating different food than they are. You may have to make your own meals separately from your family, even if you eat together. If your co-workers go out to eat at a restaurant where it's impossible to get low-calorie meals, stop going out to eat with them. When meeting your friends for dinner, just get a diet soda or coffee instead of a meal. Or if this makes you feel awkward, look up the menu online so you can decide ahead of time on a low-calorie option.

Sorry. It sucks. But it's what you have to do.

JOIN A PEER GROUP FOR ACCOUNTABILITY AND CELEBRATING VICTORIES

In the last chapter, I talked about how the people around you influence you. You can harness this for good by joining a peer group.

Find a group of people who are also trying to lose weight, and meet with each other regularly. (Ideally weekly.)

Meeting in person is nice, but if that's not practical, you can also meet by phone or online chat.

In these weekly meetings, discuss how you're doing. What wins have you had, in terms of your weight loss habits built, pounds lost, temptations resisted, clothes you're able to wear, compliments received, athletic abilities gained, all-around feeling good, etc. If you've had failures, your peers can offer you encouragement. They can remind you that losing weight is possible.

You can also use these groups for accountability - to make commitments about things you will do, and then follow up to tell them whether you kept those commitments. (But it is important not to shame yourself or other members of the group when they don't meet these commitments. You should be encouraging them that they will be able to do better next time. The group should be a positive experience.)

Peer groups like this are extremely powerful in building lasting change.

How do you start an accountability group? Simply e-mail some people you know asking if they would like to join one. An accountability group is the sort of thing that lots of people want to participate in, but few take the initiative to start. If you want more advice or step-by-step plans, google "How to start an accountability group" and you'll find dozens of people sharing their personal experiences.

While it would be best if your peer group was people trying to lose weight so that you could share specific tips, if you can't find enough people working on weight loss, you could also form a group of people trying to make other changes. Quitting smoking, quitting drinking, avoiding procrastination, etc.

WEIGH YOURSELF AT LEAST WEEKLY

You need to track your progress. This helps you to understand whether the techniques you're using are working. It also provides the positive feedback and encouragement you need for the habit to stick.

Remember: It is vitally important for you to receive a reward for your hard work. Otherwise, you will not be able to build your weight loss habit. Seeing your weight steadily drop is one of the rewards.

Weigh yourself on the same day each week. Or twice a week. (Make sure you do it at the same time each day, as your weight can fluctuate throughout the day.) And write that weight down along with the date in a notebook or spreadsheet. If you're so inclined, you can make that into a graph.

If you're doing it right, you should see your weight steadily dropping over time.

Don't expect dramatic plunges in your weight. Remember, you're making incremental small changes that you will be able to maintain for the rest of your life, and then stacking those changes on top of each other over time. This is not meant to be a fast process. It's meant to be a sustainable process.

If you're losing one to two pounds a week, you're on a good pace.

If your weight isn't dropping, or if it momentarily plateaus or even increases, don't get discouraged. This happens sometimes. Maybe you just had a bad week. Stick to the process of building healthy habits, and then once they become automatic, adding more healthy habits.

As long as you keep reducing your caloric input, your weight will keep dropping until it reaches your equilibrium weight.

USE EXTERNALLY IMPOSED COMMITMENTS

I suffer from cluster headaches, which is a condition that affects about one out of a thousand people. Every so often, I'll go into a cluster period, that lasts for about a month to six weeks, where I'll repeatedly get extremely painful headaches. Usually these headaches come in the middle of the night, but they'll also be triggered by alcohol.

I haven't seen any statistics or studies to back this up, but it's always seemed to me that someone with cluster headaches is very unlikely to be an alcoholic. When I'm in a cluster period, I'll read a bar's menu as "Would you like a cool refreshing glass of being repeatedly punched in the back of the eyeball for an hour? Only $5 during happy hour!" No thanks, I'll pass.

Telling someone "If you have this drink, you will suffer agonizing pain" is probably an effective way to get them to stop.

Cluster headaches are a natural (and somewhat extreme) version of what social scientists call a *commitment device*. This is where you set up external pressure to push you into future choices you want to make now, but are worried you won't make when the time comes. You can harness this concept to help you.

For example, you can tell your spouse, "Any time I eat more calories than I should, you get control over the TV remote for the rest of the night." If your spouse likes TV shows that you don't, that will motivate you to stick to healthy food and/or limit your portions.

You could store your high-calorie food at your neighbor's house. If you have to go over to your neighbor's and ask for it, you'll only do so if you have a good reason, and you won't eat it on a whim. (Or similarly, you could store it in a safe that your friend has the combination to.)

You could commit to putting some money in a jar every time you exceed your target calories for the day. And periodically, your spouse, kids, friend, or neighbor could use the funds in the jar to buy something they want. Or you could donate it to a worthy charity.

A couple caveats on this: You should make sure whatever methods you use either make the bad choices impossible, or involve mild hassle or embarrassment. But don't go to an extreme with something that is completely humiliating, horribly unpleasant, or that you find morally repugnant.

If you declare that every time you eat ice cream, you have to dress up like a pig and dance in the street shouting "I'm a big fat fatty," that's going to be horribly psychologically damaging, and a good way to develop an eating disorder. If you decide that any time you eat a candy bar, you have to donate $10 to the National Alliance for the Promotion of Puppy-Kicking, then you'll just end up cheating. It will be very easy to rationalize not sending that money, because why should some poor puppies suffer just because you ate a Snickers? And once you decide that, it defeats the whole purpose.

I'd also steer clear of commitments like "If I don't reach a certain weight by a certain date, I have to clean your house." You shouldn't focus on milestones, because it's detrimental to the practice of building sustainable habits. You should stick with commitments that are based on doing (or not doing) something regularly.

LOOK AT NUTRITION LABELS WHEN YOU SHOP

A theme I've tried to stress in this book is that good habits are more important than willpower. With the right habits in place, you don't *need* willpower, because healthy behavior becomes automatic.

An excellent way to put this idea into practice is to make your good decisions about what to eat at the grocery store rather than the dinner table. It's a lot easier to eat healthy when your pantry, fridge, and freezer are filled with healthy food instead of high calorie food.

But it's not always obvious what's healthy. So here's the habit you need to develop: Before you put something into your cart, flip it around to look at the nutrition label to see how many calories it is.

Then ask yourself if it's worth the calories.

I'm not saying you should never buy anything that's high calorie. I'm saying you should actively think about whether the enjoyment you will get out of eating it is worth consuming the calories, and only buy it if you make a rational decision that it is.

It's better to make that decision at the store, when you're not hungry and you don't need to rely on willpower, than when you're at home and battling the temptation to shove it all in your mouth.

You already have the habit of only buying the food that you want, or at least that you or your family plan to eat. And you probably already have the habit of checking the food's price to see if it's worth it. (If you don't, you should try to build that habit too, for the health of your bank account.) Checking the nutrition label to see if the food is worth the calories is just one more thing that you can add on to those other habits.

One important note on this is to pay attention to the listed serving size. For example, the nutrition label on pop tarts pretends that a serving is one pop tart. But does anyone ever eat *one* pop tart? No. You eat two, because that's how many are in a packet. So the box claims there's around 200 - 250 calories depending on the flavor, but you'll actually be eating 400 - 500 calories. I mean, technically there's no law saying that when you open a packet with two pop tarts, you can't put one in the toaster and the other in a Ziploc bag to go back in the box. But stop and think about whether once you see and smell that sugary goodness, you'll realistically do that.

47

UNDERSTAND SERVING SIZE

One thing that can often trip people up when trying to understand how many calories they're consuming is serving size. How much is an ounce of peanut butter? What does half a tablespoon of mayonnaise look like? Does anyone actually count the number of chips that they eat? And what if you're not eating the exact amount that the nutrition label calls a serving?

Fortunately, there's a better way, since in the modern world everyone has a calculator in their pocket.

Look at the nutrition label to see how many calories are in a serving, and how many servings per container there are. Use your phone's calculator to multiply the two together. (Or do it in your head if you're good with math.) That is how many calories there are in the whole package. (If there's only one serving or the nutrition label tells you the calories in the entire package, you can skip this step, obviously.)

Now estimate what portion of the total package you'll be eating. Divide the calories in the total package by that portion to get the calories you're eating.

For example, a bag of chips says a serving size is 13 chips, there are 9 servings per container, and a serving is 120 calories. That means the entire bag is 9 x 120 = 1,080 calories. If you're planning to eat ¼ of the bag, then you will be eating 1,080 / 4 = 270 calories.

Alternatively, you can buy things in single-serving bags/containers, which usually ends up being a bit more expensive, but saves you from having to do math and figuring out what percentage of a larger package you're eating. But make sure they actually *are* single serving. Sometimes nutrition labels will claim small containers have multiple servings. See the example from last chapter about how the label for Pop Tarts claims a packet is two servings.

NEVER EAT STRAIGHT FROM A MULTI-SERVING PACKAGE

Has this ever happened to you?

You start munching on a large bag of chips, or a box of crackers, or a large package of gummi worms, or maybe you're *trying* to be healthy and you've got a big bag of baby carrots that you're dipping in hummus. Anyway, you're eating while watching TV, or reading a book, or working, or browsing Facebook, or chatting with a friend. Then after a while, you realize you have no idea how much you just ate, but the bag seems a lot emptier, and now your stomach hurts.

Don't do that.

The most important part of the Weight Loss Habit is to think before you eat and make a conscious choice what and how much you want to consume. You can't do that if you have no clue how much you're actually eating, which is what happens when you eat straight from a multi-serving package.

There's an easy solution to this. Once you've made a conscious choice that you want to eat something that comes in a multi-serving package, decide how much you want to eat, and then pour that amount onto a plate. Then put the package away, or at least out of your reach.

Then, because you've already thought about it and made the decision, it's perfectly safe for you to mindlessly munch the amount you've predetermined should be on your plate, and you won't end up overeating.

IF YOU WILL BE DISTRACTED WHILE EATING, PREPARE YOUR PLATE WHILE NOT DISTRACTED

We're all busy people. It would be nice if we could turn eating into some sort of ritual, mindfully savoring every bite. But ain't nobody got time for that.

Let's be realistic. You spend most of your meals while watching TV. Or sitting at the computer. Or doing work. Or driving between appointments. Or at best, sitting down with your family and engaging in pleasant conversation. But not paying attention to what you're eating.

And that's totally fine. We should be spending our lives focusing on our lives, not our food. You shouldn't completely change the way you live to accommodate your diet. If you try to, your diet will inevitably fail.

The most important part of the Weight Loss Habit is to think before you eat. But it doesn't have to be *immediately* before. If you do your thinking when you're putting your food on the plate in the first place, then you don't have to pay much attention while you're eating.

You've already made a good choice and limited the calories that you have in front of you to mindlessly shove in your mouth, so you can focus on other things without having to worry.

AVOID EATING WHILE DRUNK OR ON DRUGS

When I was in college, I used to drink a tremendous amount of alcohol. I wasn't an alcoholic - I was just a college student.

I did, however, have terrible eating habits. One of my favorite things to do when drunk was to stumble down to a local takeout place and order a large cheese-fries. I'd then come back home and eat the cheese-fries, dipped in copious amounts of mayonnaise. I have no idea how many calories this was, but I'd guess somewhere between 1,000 and 1,500. (After I had already consumed a similar amount of calories of beer.)

This became such a habit that sometimes on nights I otherwise didn't have any occasion to drink, I would decide to get drunk just so I'd have an excuse to eat cheese-fries.

This isn't a book about alcohol and drug use, except insofar as most booze has a significant amount of calories. If you have a problem, I hope you seek help. But your decisions as to whether and how much alcohol and drugs to consume and the consequences of those choices are outside the scope of this book.

However, the Weight Loss Habit involves making a rational decision about what to eat. Alcohol and drugs impair your rational decision-making abilities. This is a problem.

The easiest solution to this is to just not eat while drunk or on drugs at all. Then you don't have any decisions or any figuring out to do at all. Just a hard and fast rule that you can fall back on.

This helps you avoid being like me with my cheese fries. Or being like the stereotypical stoner with the munchies. Or the trap of snacks and finger food at a party where each piece seems so small, but it all adds up to a completely unreasonable amount.

Theoretically, you could follow the advice from earlier chapters and make up a plate while you're sober. But realistically, once you finish that plate, you'll probably go back for seconds. Or dessert. Or some other snacks.

It's better and easier to just have a bright-line rule that you can remember even when impaired: No food while drunk or on drugs, period.

Now, some would argue that food is useful for absorbing the alcohol, or preventing a hangover. But water works quite well for that, and doesn't have any calories. Same with coffee, or diet soda. (Feel free to drink all the no-calorie liquids you want.)

Besides, if you're getting drunk, you're probably already consuming far more calories than you should just from the alcoholic beverages.

EAT SLOWER, AND TAKE SMALLER BITES - ESPECIALLY WHEN EATING HIGH CALORIE FOODS

You know what tastes exactly as good as a handful of M&Ms? One M&M. You know what tastes just as good as a Snickers bar? A miniature Snickers bar. You know what's even better than snarfing down an ice cream cone? Slowly licking an ice cream cone, and taking the time to enjoy it.

In an earlier chapter, I talked about finding lower calorie substitutes that were almost as tasty as high calorie foods. Taking smaller bites is a way to essentially substitute the same food for itself, but make it lower in calories. You can eat a smaller amount while tricking your taste buds into thinking you're eating the same thing.

If you eat one M&M at a time, or a smaller lick of an ice cream cone, or half a potato chip per bite instead of a whole one, you satisfy your cravings, fulfil your habitual need, and get to enjoy the taste, all while consuming fewer calories.

You can also try to slow down your eating. Instead of swallowing and taking another bite, chew for a little longer, and savor the taste. If you keep the candy in your mouth for twice as long, you can get the same enjoyment from half as much candy.

If you're just looking for something sweet, I'd suggest hard candy, since you can hold them in your mouth and continually enjoy them for a long time. One 10 calorie hard candy can last as long as two or three entire bowls of ice cream.

USE A SMALLER SPOON

Following up on the idea of taking smaller bites, here's a quick zero effort, zero willpower, zero cost way to reduce your caloric intake. (Actually, it's negative cost - it will save you money.)

Whenever you're eating something with a spoon, use the smallest spoon that is reasonable.

A small spoonful of cereal, soup, chili, or ice cream tastes exactly the same as a large spoonful. But by using a smaller spoon, you can enjoy just as many spoonfuls from a smaller amount than you would have from a larger amount if you were using a larger spoon.

You take in fewer calories, and you save money as well, since you're going through the food slower.

You can take this to a somewhat comical extreme with something like ice cream. If you're in an ice cream parlor, use one of the sample spoons to eat it. At home, use a tasting spoon or espresso spoon. (You can order sets of tasting spoons or espresso spoons on Amazon for around $7.)

USE CHEWING GUM TO KEEP YOURSELF FROM EATING

There's a hypothesis that the rise in obesity in America over the last few decades is due to smoking going out of fashion. People quit smoking and replace the vice with overeating. (Or younger people who in earlier times would have become smokers become overeaters instead.)

I'm skeptical about this completely explaining the rise in obesity. In general, I'm wary of anyone peddling a claim that there's one simple cause to an extremely complicated trend. But it's certainly plausible that the drop in smoking is one of many factors that have contributed to obesity. The simple logistical fact is that it's hard to stick food in your mouth when there's already a cigarette there.

I certainly wouldn't suggest you take up smoking in order to lose weight. Instead, you should take up smoking to look cool. (Just kidding.)

There's a way to get this weight loss benefit of smoking without all of the downsides. If you feel the need to eat out of habit, or you just want to taste something, chew some gum instead.

Like with cigarettes, you can't eat and chew gum at the same time, so chewing gum acts as a barrier to sticking food in your mouth. (This is also something you could try if you want to quit smoking.)

This is a way to hack your habit loop. When you feel the habitual craving to eat something, instead reach for gum. Then give yourself that mental pat on the back, knowing you are taking control of your own health by making good decisions.

But chewing gum won't help you look cool. You'll have to figure that part out on your own.

AVOID FILLER FOODS

For most of human history, it was a struggle to get enough calories to survive. So pretty much every civilization since the invention of agriculture has had some form of what I call "filler food."

These are things like rice, potatoes, bread, tortillas, and pasta. They are abundant, cheap, easy to grow and cook, and can be used to supplement the good stuff that people actually want to eat.

We should all be thankful these foods exist. Without them, civilization wouldn't have been able to survive. There wasn't enough good stuff to feed everyone.

But now we aren't trying to get enough calories. We're consuming too much.

If you're going to cut out calories, it's a lot easier to cut the boring stuff you don't care about instead of the food you're excited about.

Have you ever been excited to eat rice? When eating your Thai food, take a reasonable portion of the meat (or tofu), veggies, and sauce, and just skip over the rice. Same with Chinese or Mexican food.

Do potatoes even have a flavor, or do they just serve a delivery device for grease/salt/butter/sour cream/cheese/seasonings, depending on how they're cooked? So when your food comes with a side of potatoes, eat the stuff you're excited about and leave the boring old potatoes behind.

A tortilla is essentially a bag you can eat. You could instead put the contents of a burrito into a bowl and enjoy it just as much while saving 300 calories. When eating street tacos that come on two small tortillas, just eat one of the tortillas. Or just eat the contents and skip the tortillas entirely.

Bread is tasty, but you can enjoy it just as much with a thin slice as with a thick slice. So buy thinly sliced bread as an easy way to cut down on the calories in your sandwiches. Or at Subway, ask them to scoop out the sub roll so it contains less of a volume of bread. Get thin crust pizza instead of deep dish, and don't eat the ends of the crusts.

Nobody's ever excited about eating spaghetti for the sake of the spaghetti itself. It's the stuff that's mixed into the spaghetti you want. So when making a pasta dish, try using the same amount of sauce/meat/veggies/cheese/good stuff that you normally use, but less pasta. You may find that the higher good stuff to pasta ratio ends up tasting better, though there will be less volume of food.

PLAN MEALS IN ADVANCE WHEN WILLPOWER IS STRONGEST

How often has this happened to you: It's time for dinner. You look through your fridge, freezer, and pantry, trying to figure out what to eat. You know you should eat something healthy, but nothing's appealing. You get frustrated trying to figure it out, and just call Domino's instead.

As I've said before, the end of the day is when your willpower is at its lowest. Especially if you have low blood sugar. Mix in some frustration of having to make a decision where maybe you don't have the right ingredients for any healthy meal that excites you, and it becomes more and more likely that you'll make a bad choice about what to eat. And then this pattern will repeat itself every day.

It's much easier to stay healthy if you plan ahead. Try to regularly figure out what your meals will be for the next few days, and make sure you have the right ingredients for those meals. Or the premade meals in your fridge/freezer, or the time scheduled to go out to eat at a healthy restaurant you've chosen in advance. Or if you're planning to order delivery that's fine, but at least it will be a conscious rational choice you are deciding to make because it's what you actively want to do, and not a bad habit you default to out of frustration.

Then once you have that plan, you don't have that hard moment of figuring out what you want to eat and testing your willpower right when it's at its weakest. Instead, you'll have set it up such that the easiest choice and default option will be to stick with the healthy meal you planned ahead of time.

An important note about this is that you should remember to know yourself when making your plans. Do not try to punish yourself, set unrealistic standards, or plan meals that you don't like. Future you is going to be pretty much the same person as present you. If there's food you hate now, you'll still hate it in three days.

You need to plan meals that future you will *want* to eat. Otherwise, you'll just end up ignoring your plan, and that makes this whole exercise worthless. In fact, it makes it worse than useless, because you'll end up hating yourself as well as eating terribly and wasting the healthy food you leave to rot in your fridge.

So make sure to plan healthy meals you actually like.

ELIMINATE SNACKING, OR ONLY HAVE LOW-CALORIE SNACKS

One of the places where people can consume a lot of hidden calories is in snacking. You carefully practice the Weight Loss Habit when it comes to mealtimes, but your office has a bowl of candy, or nuts, or a plate of cookies, and you grab some every time you walk by.

These sneaky calories add up. It's no coincidence that the words snack and sneak sound so similar.

If you're snacking between meals, this is probably more out of habit rather than genuine hunger. And this is a habit you need to break.

Fortunately, there's a ready guide on how to do this. In Charles Duhigg's *The Power of Habit*, this is the specific example that is used on how to break a bad habit, from Duhigg's own experience. Every day around 3:00 PM he would take a break from his work, go to the office cafeteria, and get a cookie.

Duhigg set out to figure out exactly what it was that he was craving that was prompting this habit. First he tried setting an alarm for 2:30 and eating an apple, so he wouldn't be hungry at 3:00. But he still found himself craving that trip to the cafeteria for a cookie. So then he tried walking a lap around the office. But that didn't make the craving go away. Finally, he walked to the cafeteria, didn't buy a cookie, but chatted with friends for a few minutes, the way he usually would while he was eating a cookie.

He realized that it wasn't really the cookie he was craving. It was taking a break to chat with his friends. With that knowledge, it was easy for him to kick his cookie-eating habit by substituting in conversation.

So try to figure out what you're really craving when you snack. Is it a break? Then take a break to do something enjoyable other than food. Is it getting up from your desk to walk to the break room where the snacks are located? Then get up from your desk and walk around. Is it chatting with your snack buddies? Then go chat with them while not eating. Is it having the taste of something in your mouth? Then chew some gum or drink a diet soda.

The one challenge here is if you figure out that what you're craving actually is the snack itself - either from a spike in blood sugar or to fill your empty belly. In that case, what you should do is wean yourself off of it. Over a few days to weeks, start having less and less of the snack, until you are ultimately not having it at all.

Or alternatively, substitute in a different snack that is healthier. Instead of a candy bar, have an apple (Or some other fruit or low-calorie snack you enjoy). Force yourself to do that for a week or two, and it will eventually take over the habit.

THE MIRACLE OF FROZEN MEALS

There was a period of time where my wife decided to go vegan. It made her feel generally better and healthier, but she ultimately gave it up because it was just too much of a time commitment.

Every day I'd come home from work and she'd be in the kitchen blending smoothies, making pastes, sorting seeds and grains, and doing god knows what to prepare all her meals. She'd stay in the kitchen the entire evening until it was time to go to bed. Eventually she decided, "Screw this. I want my life back," and switched back to a normal diet just because it was easier.

A lot of people think this is what dieting means: You need to avoid all processed foods, so you have to freshly prepare all of your own meals. Which is fine if you love to cook, or are super-fast in the kitchen. But for the rest of us, this can be a huge barrier to losing weight.

We're busy people, and if we have to devote hours each day to meal prep, we'll end up not doing it. If we make weight loss - or any habit change - too difficult, the challenge, hassle, and time commitment makes it far more likely that we'll give up than that we'll follow through regularly enough to build the habit and succeed.

That's where frozen meals come in.

Frozen meals are the healthy eater's best friend. They tell you exactly how many calories are in them, so you can easily pick out sensible ones when you shop. There's an enormous variety so anyone can find some that they like, and have different meals throughout the week. They're quick and easy to make. All you have to do is pop them in the oven or microwave. They're inexpensive - typically between $1 and $4 a meal, depending on brands and what's on sale. And let's be honest: Most of us aren't gourmet chefs, so frozen meals are tastier than what 90% of us are capable of making.

You can shove a few weeks worth of meals into your freezer and then not have to worry about it. You can also put some in your office freezer to have healthy meals at work. If your family members or meal-mates have different dietary needs/tastes, you can each have entirely different meals without it being a hassle. Plus you don't have to deal with cleaning up the kitchen after cooking.

Also, you don't have the guilt and wasted money of buying fresh ingredients and then having to throw them away when they go bad because you never got around to using them.

The foodies and health nuts may be appalled by this advice, and scream about preservatives and processed ingredients. But whatever small hypothetical health risks there are from that stuff is dwarfed by the very real and large health problems of obesity. So ignore all that nonsense, and use this extremely easy and convenient way to reduce your calorie intake and lose weight.

EATING FAST FOOD FOR FUN AND WEIGHT LOSS

Fast food is the bogeyman of the health industry. From films like *Supersize Me* and books like *Fast Food Nation*, it's often blamed for the obesity epidemic. It's the shorthand and example of people eating terribly just because it's convenient.

Obviously, if you're regularly eating 1,200 calorie monster burgers along with a 600 calorie large fries and an extra-large 350 calorie sugary soda, then topping it off with a 1,200-calorie milkshake, that's not doing your health any favors.

All the people tut-tutting about fast food act like anyone who goes to McDonalds is a complete idiot. But there are excellent reasons to eat fast food. As its name implies, it's fast. And convenient. If you're a busy mother rushing to get your kids from school to practice to a recital to home before heading in to work at your second job, you don't have time to make a home-cooked meal.

Plus, it tastes good.

Fortunately, there are healthy ways to eat fast food. You can enjoy the convenience and flavor without downing 3,000+ calories at a meal.

First of all, get a diet soda instead of a sugary soda. That saves you a bunch of calories for free.

Next, skip the milkshakes and french fries. Yes, I know these can be delicious. But you can't expect to make fast food healthy without a bit of sacrifice.

Instead of fries, get a side-salad, which most fast food burger places will let you substitute into your meal at no extra cost. Be careful with the dressing for the salad. A lot of salad dressing is shockingly high in calories. (See the chapter on high calorie "healthy" foods.) They typically give you the same size dressing packets for the side salad as for the large salads, so try to only use a small portion of the dressing they give you.

Most fast food places have smaller burgers/items, so get one of those. They taste the same as the large marquee items - there's just less of them. So you get to enjoy the taste and convenience with fewer calories. (And as a bonus, you'll save money.)

Most fast food places also have meal salads. But make sure to get these with grilled chicken rather than crispy chicken. And again, be careful about the dressing.

If you live somewhere that requires fast food places to post their calorie contents on the menu, finding low calorie options is easy. If not, take a few minutes to go to your favorite chain's website and look at the nutritional information to pick some out.

To make things more convenient for you, I found some options at major fast food chains that are under 600 calories, and listed these in the appendix at the end of the book.

BEWARE OF HIGH CALORIE "HEALTHY" FOODS

There's a guy I know who's naturally skinny, and on top of his thin-privilege, is a health nut. He's the kind of guy who insists that processed sugar is literally poison and was terribly offended that his son's daycare occasionally gave the kids candy. Now, this is a really smart guy. (He's actually the grandson of a Nobel Prize winner.) He got a job at Google, and eschewed the sodas at the free vending machines, opting for fruit juice instead. Then after a month or two, was shocked to discover that he had gained quite a bit of weight. Why? Because fruit juice is extremely high in calories.

And that's the problem. There are a lot of foods that people think of as healthy - that Shape Magazine or Men's Health or Buzzfeed or food gurus tell you that you should eat - which are extremely high in calories. These can be a huge pitfall if you're trying to monitor your calories in order to lose weight.

Just to be clear, I'm not saying you shouldn't eat these foods. Just that you shouldn't go nuts and assume that because they're "healthy" it's okay to eat as much as you want. You still need to pay attention to calories and portion size, and most importantly, think before you eat. In other words, still practice the Weight Loss Habit even with "healthy" food.

Except for celery. You can eat as much of that as you want, so feel free to abandon all moderation there. As long as you're not dipping it in anything or putting something on top.

Here are some foods to be wary of:

[Note: Calorie counts here are approximate, based on representative versions of these. They may vary slightly from product to product.]

Fruit Juice: Apple juice, orange juice, and cranberry juice all have 110 calories per 8 ounce serving. That's more calories per ounce than Coke. Note that Tropicana makes Trop50 orange juice that only has 50 calories, which is an improvement, though you still shouldn't go nuts with it. Ocean Spray has a line of 5 calorie cranberry juice cocktails that are okay to go nuts with.

Nuts: Speaking of nuts, there's 170 calories in every ounce of peanuts. (And if you're eating peanuts, you'll probably have several ounces.) Or 11 calories per peanut. There are 165 calories in an ounce of almonds. There are 185 calories in an ounce of walnuts. 195 calories in an ounce of pecans. 160 calories in an ounce of pistachios.

Peanut Butter: A serving size of peanut butter is listed as 2 tablespoons, which is 190 calories. But realistically, a sandwich-worth is at least double that.

Dried Fruit: An apricot is a healthy low-calorie snack that's less than 20 calories. Twenty apricots, on the other hand, is not such a healthy snack. That's what you're eating when you mindlessly munch dried fruit. The calories don't go away when the fruit dries out, but it does make it a lot easier to eat way too much. In fact, dried fruit often has added sugar, making it higher in calories than the original fruit.

Pita Bread: Pita is just a denser form of bread. That doesn't make it healthier. One pita has 165 calories.

Hummus: Two ounces of hummus, which is the size of a Sabra single-serving cup, has 150 calories. And if you're eating your hummus from a larger container, you'll likely have far more than that.

Hummus and Pita: Basic addition here. One pita and a single-serving cup of hummus are 315 calories. Two pita and four ounces of hummus are 630 calories. Three pita and six ounces of hummus are 945 calories. This quickly adds up.

Avocados: An avocado has about 325 calories. Yes, people will tell you that it's good fat, and heart healthy, and I'll tell you it's delicious. It's still a lot of calories.

Restaurant Salads: Lettuce is low in calories, so it's natural to think that a salad which is mostly lettuce must be low in calories. But while a salad is *mostly* lettuce, often that remainder is very high in calories - enough to render the whole thing unhealthy. For example, the Chili's Santa Fe Chicken Salad is 940 calories, the Boneless Buffalo Chicken Salad is 1020, and the Quesadilla Explosion Salad is a whopping 1410 calories. Okay, maybe you're not foolish enough to think that something with "Quesadilla Explosion" in its name is going to be healthy. But the California Pizza Kitchen Thai Crunch salad with avocado is 1290 calories, the Waldorf Chicken salad is 1320 calories, the BBQ Chicken Chopped Salad with Mustard Herb Vinaigrette dressing is 1350 calories. Even the Roasted Veggie salad can be up to 830 calories depending on the dressing you get.

Salad Dressing: A lot of salad dressings have a shocking amount of calories, stemming from their high fat or sugar content. Be very careful to check the nutrition labels. Look for the low-cal/low-fat versions, even though they aren't as tasty. Aim for dressings that are 35 calories or less/per listed serving. And remember that what they call a serving is probably a lot less than you'll actually use. Though if you can start eating your salads with less dressing, that's an improvement.

Vegetables dipped in stuff: Carrots, celery, zucchini, etc. are great. But when you dip them in peanut butter, cream cheese, ranch dip, etc., usually the things you're dipping them in have a lot of calories, and you have no idea how much you're consuming.

Sports Drinks: The sports drinks' marketing tries to convince you that it's vital to consume their product in order to replenish your precious bodily fluids after exercise. However you can also replenish your fluids with water, which is zero calories and free. As for all the other stuff in sports drinks, you're not an elite athlete and you don't need it. If you really really want it, Gatorade and Powerade both make zero/low calorie versions, so buy those.

Vegan, Gluten-Free, and Paleo Foods: Oreos are vegan. Ice cream is gluten-free. And technically, a five-gallon bucket of pure lard is paleo. Just because something fits into one of these diets doesn't make it healthy. If you go to Veggie Grill and get their Nashville Hot Chickin' Sandwich with a side of Sweetheart Fries. That's 1,270 calories. Add in some 110 calorie ranch dressing to dip your Sweetheart Fries in, a 270 calorie Pineapple Ginger Beet Agua Fresca to drink and a 550 calorie Choco-Churro Sundae for dessert, and your lunch at the "healthy" vegetarian restaurant is 2,200 calories.

Dark Chocolate: A trendy piece of food advice is to eat dark chocolate, because it's supposed to be healthy, for, uh, reasons. A bar of Hershey's Special Dark has 200 calories, which is only 20 fewer than a regular Hershey bar. If you're only having a 1/12 bar piece each day, that's 17 calories, which isn't a big deal. But if you're having a whole bar or even half a bar a day, that 200 or 100 daily calories will add up.

Milk, Non-Fat Milk, and Milk Substitutes: It does a body good. It also does a body 160 calories per 8 ounce serving. You can switch to skim milk to reduce calories, but it doesn't eliminate them. Skim milk is still 90 calories per 8 ounce serving, which is more calories per ounce than sugary soda. Almond milk is still 60 calories per 8 ounces (or 80 calories for vanilla almond milk). If you get unsweetened almond milk, then you're getting down to 30 calories, which is in the range where you don't have to worry so much. And remember to pay attention to portion size. All these numbers are per eight ounces or one cup. If you drink more, you have to multiply appropriately.

Frozen Yogurt: Many people think of frozen yogurt as a healthier alternative to ice cream. But it is often loaded with calories. In many cases, even more so than ice cream. Especially when you start mixing in toppings. You can try to get the sugar-free yogurt, and mix in fruit instead of Nutella/cookies to limit the calories. But even so, check the nutrition info and make sure you understand what you're eating.

Regular Yogurt: Yogurt is loaded with probiotics, which the health nuts insist is good. But a lot of yogurt is loaded with calories as well. It's typically around 150 calories per serving, but some flavors can get up to 300 calories, while light yogurt is usually more like 90 calories.

Granola Bars, NutriGrain Bars, and Protein Bars: Protein bars, power bars, Clif bars, etc., are usually in the neighborhood of 250 - 300 calories. That's okay as a meal replacement, but not as a snack or part of a meal. Granola bars and NutriGrain bars are in the 100 - 150 calorie range.

Cole Slaw: It's shredded cabbage. It must be healthy, right? Not when it's mixed with a bunch of mayonnaise and sugar. Check the nutrition label. It's shockingly high in calories. (The exact amount will depend on the specific brand/recipe.)

Wheat Bread: Just because it uses 100% whole grains doesn't mean the calories go away. Each slice of Oroweat 100% Whole Wheat Bread has 90 calories.

Bagels: It's breakfast time, and someone brought in donuts. You decide you'll be healthy and have a bagel instead. Nope. Bagels typically have as many or more calories as donuts. About 250 to 350, depending on the size, type, and density. Add another 100 calories or more if you put cream cheese on it.

Bran Muffins: Presumably you already know muffins are high in calories. That doesn't change if you add "Bran" into their name. Since there's no standard size of a muffin I can't tell you exactly how many calories, but it's probably between 300 and 600.

Smoothies: Smoothies can be all over the map, depending on how they're made. If they're mostly fruit and vegetables, they're usually fairly low in calories, especially if you're having them as a meal replacement. And obviously the size makes a huge difference. A small McDonalds strawberry-banana smoothie is only 190 calories. On the other hand, if they're filled with ice cream or high-fat yogurt, peanut butter, Nutella, honey, and other calorie-dense foods, they can be incredibly bad for you. A large Jamba Juice Peanut Butter Moo'd is 910 calories.

Beyond/Impossible Meat: If you're a vegetarian for moral, ethical, or environmentalist reasons, or just because it makes you feel better, Beyond Meat and Impossible Meat are fine choices. But they won't help you cut calories. The Carl's Jr Beyond Famous Star With Cheese is 40 *more* calories than the regular Famous Star With Cheese.

Honey: Honey is an all-natural sugar substitute. It's delicious, unprocessed, and comes straight from a bee's butt. (Or is it mouth? Honey-udders? No, I'm pretty sure that's wrong. Okay, full disclosure. I don't actually know how bees make honey.) Anyway, the point is that while it may be all natural and unprocessed, it is not a *low-calorie* sugar substitute. There's 60 calories per serving of honey.

Rice (including whole grain and brown rice): Some people have the idea that rice is healthy. I guess because it's bland and unenjoyable to eat. But it has 205 calories per cup of white rice or 215 calories per cup of brown or whole grain rice, and you'll probably end up eating a lot more than a cup if you aren't careful. If you've ever eaten too much Chinese, Japanese, or Thai food, and then been laying around clutching your belly and regretting your life choices, excessive rice was probably the culprit. (Unless it was too many noodles, but you already knew they weren't healthy.) Note that you can save a huge amount of calories by switching to cauliflower rice, which is only 25 calories per cup.

LEARN HOW MANY CALORIES ARE IN YOUR FAVORITE FOODS - ESPECIALLY AT RESTAURANTS

In the last few chapters, I talked about some horrible options to eat at Veggie Grill, Chili's, CPK, and Jamba Juice, and some good options to eat at fast food places. (See appendix for specific fast food recommendations.)

You should get into the habit of finding this information out on your own.

For food you buy in a store, you can just check the nutrition labels. And if you live somewhere that restaurants are required to post calorie counts, you can check at the restaurant. But if you live elsewhere, you have to do a bit of research.

Fortunately, we live in an age where this research is easy. Simply google "Name of restaurant" and "nutrition information." You should find the information on the restaurant's own website, or alternatively, tons of other sources have compiled the information as well.

You may find it helpful to take notes of the calorie counts for the specific items you order or may order in the future. And don't forget that sometimes they'll be sneaky on their website. Check the size (Is this the small or the large) and make sure it includes things like condiments, salad dressings, sides, etc. Or else add the calorie count for those in.

I live somewhere that restaurants post calorie counts, but I still like to check the website nutrition information ahead of time, so that I can plan out a rational informed choice rather than making a snap decision on the spot.

Over time, you should start to learn/memorize the specific counts of the foods you eat the most, which will make this process much easier.

And remember, you don't have to eat the entire meal. You can take half the meal home, or leave some on the plate. But it's better if you order something lower in calories in the first place, so you don't have to rely on willpower once you've started eating.

PAY ATTENTION TO HOW YOU FEEL AFTER YOU EAT

Start trying to pay attention to how your body and mind feel after you eat.

I don't mean that you should do some sort of elaborate body scan meditation, or consistently keep a food journal. That's too much work, and realistically, you're not going to do it.

What I mean is, maybe a half hour to an hour after you finish eating, pause for a second to ask yourself, "How does my stomach feel, what's my energy level like, and what is my mood?"

If any of those are better or worse than is normal for you, think about what you ate, and whether it could be related to what you're feeling.

Also, when you poop, if things are going abnormally well or poorly, think about your recent food and whether it could be related.

If you start to notice a consistent pattern between certain foods and how you feel, take the next step, which involves a little bit of mental acrobatics:

You need to shift your mindset to incorporate the way the food makes you feel into your idea of how much you "like" the food.

For example, I have noticed that creamy pasta dishes make me feel run down and low energy. So while I enjoy the *flavor* of creamy pasta dishes, I don't *like* creamy pasta dishes, because the totality of the experience of eating them is unpleasant.

Eating a creamy pasta dish means not just enjoying something delicious, but also feeling crappy afterward. Since I don't want to feel crappy, I don't want the creamy pasta dish in the first place.

(Don't worry. I know you don't want to hear about which foods affect my poop. That's all I'm going to say about that.)

This is a useful mental shift, because usually the foods that make you feel bad are the foods that are high in calories, and cutting them out will help you lose weight. So realizing that you don't *want* to eat them helps to eliminate the temptation, and makes it far easier to eat lower-calorie foods instead.

74

USE VISUAL PATTERN MATCHING GAMES AS DISTRACTIONS

Sometimes you have a craving that you know is a bad idea. You're applying the Weight Loss Habit, rationally thinking about it, and deciding you shouldn't eat it. But you can't shake the craving. The craving is a continual drain against your willpower, and you worry you'll eventually give in and eat the food you know you shouldn't. Even if you fight it off, the craving is an annoying distraction, and reduces the willpower you have available for other things.

There's an easy way to fight this: Play visual pattern matching games like Candy Crush, Tetris, Bejeweled, Set, or a jigsaw puzzle.

It sounds weird, but this works. Because humans evolved with vision as their primary sense, a large portion of the human brain is dedicated to processing visual information. When you play a visual pattern matching game, the challenging visuospatial task crowds out all other thoughts.

This is why games like Candy Crush are so addictive. You can harness this power for good, by using the way the human brain is designed to wipe out unhelpful cravings.

As a side note, this trick is also useful for fighting anxiety and staving off panic attacks.

PAY ATTENTION TO CRAVINGS THAT AREN'T BAD IDEAS

You'll often get a craving for something that you know is unhealthy: Ice cream, or pizza, or an entire bucket of gummy worms. Since you have common sense, you know these are bad ideas. So you can rationally decide to ignore the craving. (Or rationally decide it is worth indulging it with moderation, which is also okay.)

And sometimes you'll get cravings for things that aren't particularly unhealthy or high-calorie. This will especially be the case as you pick up more and more of the habits in this book, and are consuming fewer and fewer calories.

For example, you may suddenly decide you really want gefilte fish. Or kimchi. Or tomato soup.

Pay attention to these latter kinds of cravings.

It may be that as you've reduced your caloric intake, you've cut out some vital nutrients you need. And this is your body's way of telling you it needs something. So when the craving isn't for a high-calorie junk food, you should indulge it.

Plus, it's a good way to feel like you're giving yourself a treat, without being unhealthy and consuming a lot of calories.

HAVE A SMALL SNACK OR NOTHING FOR BREAKFAST

They say, "breakfast is the most important meal of the day." Who are *they*? I don't know. The people who say breakfast is the most important meal of the day. Why is breakfast so important? I don't know. Because *they* say so.

One of the quickest ways to cut a large number of calories from your daily consumption is to drop from three meals to two. Especially if you've been having a high calorie breakfast that includes pancakes, muffins, rolls, juice, sausage, etc.

Try skipping breakfast, and see how you feel. It may be that you're eating breakfast out of habit, and not because you need it.

Everyone's body is different. Some people do need to eat something in the morning to feel decent. But usually they don't need a massive meal. If this is you, try having a small snack, like an apple or granola bar. Something under 200 calories.

You could also try gradually reducing the size of your breakfast over time. Remember that incremental changes are much easier than a sudden shock. So drop from three pancakes to two, then after a week only have one, then the next week have no pancakes.

NEVER HAVE TWO BIG MEALS IN A ROW

Sometimes you make the intentional decision that a high calorie meal is worth it, and that's okay. And sometimes you slip up and eat a high calorie meal without thinking about it. That's not ideal, but all you can do is try to do better moving forward.

Then you come to the next meal. You're still digesting the large meal you had earlier. Having *another* large meal is almost certainly not going to be a good decision. You won't enjoy it much. You'll end up hurting your stomach. You risk breaking all your hard-built habits.

So it's best to just have a hard and fast rule so you don't even have to think about it: Never eat two big meals in a row. If you had a big meal for lunch, have a small dinner. If you had a big meal for dinner, have a small meal for lunch the next day. (And also follow the advice about skipping breakfast.)

Or if you have an extremely large meal, you could consider skipping the next meal entirely. If you're not hungry at all, don't eat. Though you should exercise caution with this if you're also skipping breakfast. You don't want to leave yourself so famished that you end up having a huge meal the next time you eat, and then repeat the cycle. It may be better to have a small snack so you avoid this. But it may not. You should know yourself and learn how your cravings work. Remember, ultimately you want to be in control of your hunger, rather than having your hunger be in control of you.

You should also think about this rule in a forward-looking way. When deciding what to eat, consider your next meal. If you know your next meal is likely to be large, make sure to have a small meal now. So you can make the rational decision to have a light lunch (or no lunch) the day of Thanksgiving, or a small dinner the night before that big Mother's Day brunch.

CHANGE GROCERY STORES TO CHANGE BUYING HABITS

The easiest way to avoid eating high-calorie/junk food is to not buy it in the first place. But sometimes, when you're shopping, your habits take over and you buy food without meaning to.

You want to build the habit of thinking before you buy food. If this proves difficult, you can give yourself a little help by changing grocery stores. That will disrupt your existing buying habits.

That way, you won't be able to make your usual purchases on autopilot. You'll already have to think before you buy things, if only to figure out where they are in an unfamiliar store. That will give you the opportunity to also think about whether you should be buying the particular item at all.

This isn't for everyone. But if you struggle with the kinds of foods you buy, try this out to give yourself a little help.

USE LITTLE NUDGES TO MAKE GOOD HABITS EASIER AND BAD HABITS HARDER

Remember that one of the guiding principles of the Weight Loss Habit is to make losing weight as easy as possible. In that spirit, you should arrange your life to make good decisions easier, and bad decisions harder.

Sometimes little nudges make a big difference. There's a lot of truth to the saying, "Out of sight, out of mind." So make sure healthy stuff is in sight, and unhealthy stuff is out of sight. And the healthy stuff is convenient, while the unhealthy stuff is inconvenient.

Put fruit in a bowl on your table, and the candy in the back of a cabinet. (Or locked in a safe. Or don't buy candy at all.)

Put your running shoes next to your bed.

Delete the Dominos app from your phone, and log out from their website, so ordering is more of a hassle.

Buy food in single serving packages. Or when you buy food in multi-serving packages that you're likely to munch too much of, portion it out yourself into single serving Ziploc bags, so when you're hungry you can just grab the right amount.

Don't keep junk food in the house at all, so when you decide to have it, you have to make the effort to go out and buy it.

Keep your exercise gear out and ready to use.

See if you can come up with your own ideas to nudge yourself in positive directions.

AVOID BUFFETS

In the vein of using little nudges to make good decisions easier and bad decisions harder, buffets are a place where bad decisions are incredibly easy and good decisions are extremely hard. It's best to avoid this situation by not going to buffets at all.

You should be fostering the habit of eating smaller amounts of food. Whereas at buffets, everything is screaming at you to eat **all of the food, all at once.**

Even if you're trying to make good decisions, you'll end up taking a little bit of this, and a little bit of that, and a little of this other thing, and before you know it your plate will be full and there will still be three more stations you want to check out when you get seconds, and that's not even touching on dessert.

And of course, you have no idea how many calories are in any of the stuff you're eating. But it's probably a lot.

Sometimes buffets can't be avoided. You can make the decision not to go to Golden Corral, but maybe you'll be at a wedding where the food is served buffet-style. Or maybe all your friends want to go to a buffet and you feel like you can't avoid that social pressure. How do you handle this?

First, you should take a lap where you review the available food, without a plate in your hand so you aren't tempted to take anything. Your goal is to identify a few things:

- What are the foods you're most excited about?
- What are some low-calorie but filling foods, such as vegetables?
- What are some high-calorie foods that are not very exciting or that you could get all the time, which you should avoid? Such as pizza, french fries, rolls/bread, and ice cream?

Now that you've gathered information, you can think about what you should eat, and make a plan. Decide what and how much of the exciting foods to take, mixed with the low-calorie foods. Plan not to take any of the high-calorie and not-exciting or could-get-all-the-time foods. Before you go back with a plate, know what you are going to take. Make sure any potential desserts you may want are included in this plan.

Then when you go back, make sure you take a smaller plate if it's offered. And stick to the plan that you rationally decided on.

Once you finish that plate, think really really hard about whether it's a good idea to get seconds, or to get desserts that weren't already part of your plan. (On the other hand, it's perfectly fine to decide *not* to get a dessert that you had originally planned to get, if you realize you're no longer hungry for it.)

It's also very important to shake yourself of the mentality that you need to "get your money's worth" from the buffet. Don't think of it as paying to eat as much food as possible. You are paying so that you can eat the optimal amount of food to promote your long-term health and happiness, which is going to be far less than the amount of food you can physically shove into your stomach. (Though this is another reason to avoid buffets - especially expensive ones. When you aren't eating a huge amount, you can usually find better food for less money elsewhere.)

THINK OF TAKEOUT OR DELIVERY AS MULTIPLE MEALS

A lot of restaurant meals contain far too many calories. Especially if you're someone with a slow metabolism who should be consuming fewer calories than the average person.

But they're so delicious, and we want to eat them. And take-out and delivery are so convenient for our busy lives.

I mentioned before that it can feel weird and awkward to immediately put half your meal in a take-home container when you're at a restaurant. But this isn't the case when you're *already home*.

When you order larger meals for home, think of them as multiple meals. "This pizza is my dinner and my lunch for tomorrow." "This Chinese takeout is my dinner for the next three days."

Have this plan in mind in a forward-thinking way. If you know that what you're eating is supposed to be your meal for tomorrow, you're much more likely to stop eating partway through. You can make this even easier for yourself by dividing it up in advance and only putting the single meal's portion on your plate.

IT'S ALL ONE SESSION - NO CHEAT DAYS

There's a saying that professional poker players have: "It's all one session."

They don't want to get overly concerned with whether they are winning or losing on a particular day or in one single tournament. What matters is how much they are winning over their entire career.

You should apply the same way of thinking to your weight loss. Your calorie count does not reset every day. It's a running total throughout your life.

One of the many reasons traditional diets fail is that people often try to insert a loophole by including a "cheat day." But calling it a cheat day doesn't make the calories disappear. (And I have some additional bad news: The "I'm eating it off someone else's plate" loophole doesn't work either.)

When a diet is based on deprivation and self-flagellation, it's natural to want to rebel against it by pretending there are days where you're allowed to pig out. But with the Weight Loss Habit, where you're allowed to eat food you enjoy when you make the rational decision to do so (as long as you don't eat too much of it), this shouldn't be necessary.

There may be special occasions when you make the rational decision to turn your brain off and just enjoy yourself. On your birthday, or Christmas, or if you're taking a trip to Disneyland, or if you're making a once-in-a-lifetime visit to a fancy schmancy gourmet restaurant. And that's fine, as long as it's extremely rare. But these special occasions should be no more than a few times a year, and not "Because it's Tuesday."

THINK OF YOURSELF IN THE THIRD PERSON TO MAKE BETTER DECISIONS

If you find yourself struggling to make good decisions, try thinking about yourself in the third person. Instead of asking yourself, "Should I eat this," ask "Should Jane eat this?" (Assuming Jane is your name. If Jane is some random woman you don't know, this won't be particularly helpful.)

It sounds silly, but this has been proven to give you a bit of emotional distance, which helps you make better decisions.

SOME FOODS YOU SHOULD AVOID

Throughout this book, I've been saying it's okay to eat what you want, as long as you do it with moderation and only eat unhealthy food when you've thought about it and made the rational decision that doing so is a good idea. But there are some particular foods that are almost always a bad idea and I highly recommend you steer clear of.

Milkshakes: Milkshakes are just a method for consuming huge amounts of ice cream quickly. They have an astounding amount of calories. They're an excellent way to consume 1000+ calories in 90 seconds. If you're really craving a milkshake, have ice cream instead. You'll probably enjoy it more, and consume fewer calories.

French Fries: French fries add a huge amount of calories to your meal, and they usually are an afterthought to what you enjoy. They're the difference between fast food being relatively healthy and fast food being fat food.

Restaurant bread and rolls: The bread and rolls they serve in restaurants are typically 200 - 300 calories per piece, and they're easy to eat mindlessly. You down a few of them, and you've already eaten way too much before your meal even arrives.

Restaurant tortilla chips: These are even worse than bread and rolls, because they contain a shocking amount of calories, and you generally have no idea how many of them you're eating. You just munch away until the basket is empty, and then ask them to bring another one. Don't do that.

Cheesecake: They are incredibly dense with calories. Especially at restaurants.

Outback Steakhouse Bloomin' Onion: Just don't.

FORTY-FIVE WAYS TO EXERCISE THAT AREN'T GOING TO THE GYM

Up until now, I've focused on eating habits rather than exercise, because diet has a much bigger impact on your weight and overall health. But exercise certainly has *some* impact. And you absolutely should be getting exercise.

But not at the gym. Here's the dirty little secret about the gym industry: **Gyms are only for people who enjoy going to the gym.** Take note of that. Commit it to memory. Recall it anytime a commercial, salesperson, corporate wellness program, overeager gym cultist, New Year's Resolution bug, doctor, or well-meaning friend suggests you join one. **Do not join a gym unless you are the kind of person who finds the gym fun.** If you force yourself to join a gym when you aren't a gym-lover, you are just wasting your money, and setting yourself up for frustration, failure, and self-hatred.

There's a reason gyms offer huge discounts to people willing to make long-term commitments. They aren't in the business of making less money when they could be making more money. They know the vast majority of people who sign up will end up hating it, and stop coming after a few sessions. Then they'll be collecting your money in exchange for nothing but your own self-guilt.

And let's face it. Gyms suck. You've got to take a bunch of time out of your busy day to fight traffic, then be in a hot sweaty room with a bunch of people in better shape than you judging you while you try to figure out complicated equipment. You get harassed by personal trainers eager for your hard-earned cash. If you're a woman, you have to deal with creepy dudes trying to creep on you, and if you're a man, you have to deal with old naked creepy dudes in the locker room trying to have conversations with you while their dongs flap around in your face. (And why *do* old men wander around gym locker rooms with their bits waving all over? I've never been able to figure that out.) All while bad music plays loudly.

For some people, the gym is enjoyable enough that they're willing to put up with all that. That's great for them. People who love the gym should absolutely keep going, and I'm happy for them that businesses exist to provide the services they are willing to pay for.

However that doesn't describe those of us who know the Struggle. Gyms aren't for us. So don't join one. But do get exercise.

You've probably tried to start an exercise routine in the past, but haven't kept it up. Even if it didn't involve a gym, you fell off the wagon. Or perhaps, climbed on the wagon and had someone pull you so you didn't have to walk. The reason you didn't keep it up was because you didn't like it. You were relying on willpower, and willpower isn't enough. Once your initial enthusiasm faded, your busy day took precedence, and you stopped doing it.

Why will it be different this time? Here is the trick:

Your exercise routine needs to be something that is easy and convenient, or even better, enjoyable.

If it's easy and convenient, then it takes far less willpower. And if it's fun, then you're excited to do it and it takes no willpower at all.

So here are a whole bunch of easy, convenient, and/or fun ways that out of shape people who don't like the gym can get some exercise:

1. **Buy a treadmill, stationary bike, or elliptical machine, and use them while watching TV.**

2. **Run in place while watching TV.** It's cheaper than buying equipment.

3. **Walk back and forth while watching TV.** If you don't like running. My mother does this. She takes 10,000 steps a day to satisfy the demands of her fitness tracker without leaving her living room.

4. **Get a treadmill desk so you can walk while working, Facebooking, surfing the web, etc.**

5. **Lift weights at home.** Just make sure you do the kind of lifting where you don't need a spotter.

6. **Lift homemade weights at home.** You can find plenty of instructions online for cheap weight substitutes and workouts you can do without spending the money on an expensive weight kit. Milk jugs filled with water, and things like that.

7. **Jumping jacks, pushups, sit-ups, and other calisthenics.**

8. **Walk your dog.** If you don't have a dog, you can borrow one from a friend or neighbor. Or volunteer at a local animal shelter, which will have the added bonus of feeling proud about doing a good deed. Or sign up with a dog-walking service like Wag, and make some extra money.

9. **Jog with your dog.** Your dog will probably enjoy it.

10. **Take a nice walk in the park with a loved one.**

11. **Go hiking with loved ones or friends.** With great views and enjoyable conversations, you won't even notice that you're working out.

12. **Go swimming.** I'm not talking about swimming laps using proper technique. Just frolicking around in a pool, ocean, or lake is a lot more fun, and still burns plenty of calories. If you don't have your own pool, ask around to find if a friend will let you use theirs. Your community may have a public pool as well.

13. **Go boogie boarding.** Taking up surfing is unrealistic, because you have to be in really good shape. But wading out to jump on a boogie board is something most people can do.

14. **Go skiing or snowboarding.**

15. **Play a one-on-one sport with a friend/loved one.** You can either find someone in similar shape and at the same skill level as you, or find someone who is better than you and accept that you'll lose a lot. It's okay to lose when the goal is to get exercise and have fun. This is what I did when I was first shedding off the pounds. I had a weekly racquetball session with my roommate. He had Thin Privilege, and could run circles around me. (Not quite literally - I was fat and those were some big circles.) But I didn't mind, because it was fun. And when I finally won a game, after months of losing, it was extremely satisfying.

16. **Join a sports league.** If you're embarrassed or feel like you wouldn't be welcome in a league where your skill and stamina level is far below average, start your own. Call it the "Overweight and Out of Shape Basketball League" (or

whatever sport) and recruit friends, or post on Meetup, Nextdoor, Facebook, flyers in coffee shops, your church newsletter, etc., to find others who are interested.

17. **Start a "Weird Sports League."** Either with your friends, or with strangers. Google for rules to obscure sports, and try them out. Since everybody's new to them, nobody will be good, and you won't have to be embarrassed about your lack of skill.

18. **Take a fun bike ride.**

19. **Ride your bike to work.** This isn't practical for a lot of people, but it might be for you.

20. **Walk a few extra bus/train/subway stops during your commute.**

21. **Take the stairs instead of the elevator to your office or apartment.**

22. **Play with your kids.**

23. **Take up a martial art.** Usually people start martial arts as children, but there's no law saying you can't do it as an overweight adult. Martial arts instructors tend to be fairly direct people. Call around and ask them if it would make sense for you, until you find one who says it would.

24. **Join a CrossFit cult.** Okay, I admit this is kind of like a gym. And a lot of crossfitters tend to be quite intense and intimidating. But some CrossFit clubs are very welcoming and supportive of newbies. If you find one of those, it can be an extremely positive experience. And as a bonus, you'll make a lot of new friends. This isn't for everyone, but I have several friends that love it.

25. **Yoga.** Maybe not at a studio, but there are a gajillion YouTube videos and apps for beginners.

26. **Play golf.**

27. **Go dancing.** Or dance in your own home.

28. **Play a dance-based video game, or another video game that involves physical movement.**

29. **Put on music and dance/rock out while cleaning and doing your regular weekly chores.**

30. **Get a membership at a zoo, museum, botanical garden, etc. that you can enjoy weekly walks through.**

I asked people on my blog for suggestions, and here are some they came up with:

31. **Use your lunch break at work to walk, either up and down stairs or around the block.** *- Submitted by Rose Meiri*

32. **Play augmented reality games such as Pokemon Go or Wizards United that get you out walking in the real world. And consider running between your goals.** *- Submitted by Rose Meiri*

33. **Walk to the grocery store, or any errand that is under a mile away and involves purchases that can be fit in a backpack.** *- Submitted by Rae Majka*

34. **Get an annual pass to a nearby theme park, and you'll spend plenty of time walking around. (Make sure you don't buy the high-calorie snacks though.)** *- Submitted by Nate Wolff*

35. **Walk around the mall, or Costco, or some other large store or place that has interesting stuff.** Just make sure you don't sample all the food. *- Submitted by Nate Wolff*

36. **Play an "exercise game" similar to a drinking game. Every time a character on TV says a certain phrase or does a certain thing, do five push-ups, or sit-ups, or jumping jacks, or the exercise of your choice.** *- Submitted by Nate Wolff*

37. **Use the exercise stations in the park. See if you can find some you enjoy.** *- Submitted by Nate Wolff*

38. **Take the farthest possible parking space from where you are going.** *- Submitted by Nate Wolff*

39. **Take a walk whenever you're on long phone calls - especially work conference calls.** *- Submitted by Nate Wolff*

40. **Geocaching, which is like hiking but you use GPS to try to find hidden items.** *- Submitted by Rose Meiri*

41. **Carry your baby/toddler while doing chores.** *- Submitted by Rae Majka*

42. **Go roller skating, which is a lot of fun.** *- Submitted by Crystal Jean Baranyk*

43. **Get your kids hooked on some sort of fun exercise program like GoNoodle, and play along with them.** *- Submitted by Rae Majka*

44. **Do some volunteer work with programs like Big Brothers/Big Sisters that will make you keep up with an active child, at a zoo or hospital that will keep you on your feet, or that involves physical work like highway cleanups and sorting clothes for the homeless.** *- Submitted by Thea Rivera*

45. **Wear ankle and wrist weights as you go about your day.** *- Submitted by Sheila Friedman*

EXERCISE AT THE SAME TIME EACH WEEK

In the last chapter, I laid out a bunch of ways to make exercise fun, easy, and/or convenient. Or at least, not too much of a burden.

The important thing with these methods of exercise is to make them into a habit. They aren't going to do you any good if you try them once and then forget about them. Exercise needs to be consistent.

If the exercise is something you actively enjoy, this may not be too difficult. The same if it is something you're forced to do. You're going to walk your dog twice a day no matter what. But what about the exercises that are small burdens?

Here we run into the same problem that exists with traditional diets. You'll tend to do them a few times when you have that initial motivation, but once that fades, your busy schedule and natural inertia will take over, and they'll fall by the wayside.

How do you combat that?

The trick is to make it into a consistent schedule. Don't just say, "I'll run on the treadmill in front of my TV when I can find the time." Say "I'll run on the treadmill in front of my TV every Monday and Thursday at 7:00 AM." And then put it on your calendar.

It's that consistency of doing it at the same time every week that turns it into a habit. Schedule it, and actually follow through with that schedule. Eventually, it will become automatic.

Gretchen Rubin, the self-help guru and author of Better Than Before that I've mentioned earlier, likes to say, "Something that can be done at any time is often done at no time." So don't assume you'll exercise at any time. Exercise at a specific planned time.

Another nice benefit of scheduling your exercise is that it relieves you of a sense of guilt when you're *not* exercising. You can flop on the couch in the evening, and you don't have that lingering voice in your head saying,

"Maybe I should be exercising." Because you know the specific times that you *should* be exercising, and have the confidence in yourself that you will exercise at those times.

94

REWARD YOURSELF DURING OR AFTER EXERCISE (BUT NOT WITH FOOD)

Remember my tip about forming habits from Part 1: To be able to form a habit, it's really best if it's something that's easy, convenient, enjoyable, provides immediate positive feedback, or is incremental improvements over time.

You can kind of cheat this with exercise, by making it more enjoyable and giving yourself immediate positive feedback through the use of a reward.

If you do something that makes you happy or is really enjoyable immediately after, or even better - during - exercise, then you'll mentally associate the two things, and start to crave exercise because of the reward.

Some possible rewards are:

- **Watch a favorite or "guilty pleasure" TV show.**

- **Watch movies.**

- **Exercise with friends so that you can socialize at the same time.**

- **Listen to your favorite music.**

- **Listen to your favorite podcast.**

- **Get a massage.**

- **Take a relaxing hot shower.**

- **Take a relaxing bath.**

- **Chill out in the hot tub.**

- **Play your favorite video game.**

- **Take in pleasant scenery.** (During a walk, hike, jog, or bike-ride.)

- **Window-shop or look at interesting stuff during a walk through a mall, museum, zoo, library, etc.**

- **Read a beloved book.**

- **Do a crossword puzzle.**

- **Watch stand-up comedy.**

- **Watch YouTube videos.**

- **Play/snuggle with your pets.**

- **Play/snuggle with your children.**

- **Take a nap.**

- **Sexy time with your partner.** (Obviously only if your partner is down for this, and they'd probably prefer if you take a shower first.)

- **Sexy time with yourself.**

Pick whichever one of these suits you best, or come up with your own.

However, one reward you *shouldn't* use is any sort of food. This is counterproductive. You don't want to undo all the good work you did burning calories through your exercise by consuming a high-calorie food.

But more importantly, you don't want to build the habit of seeing food as a reward. As someone following the Weight Loss Habit, this is undercutting the mentality you need to foster.

Besides, the world offers an incredibly array of joyous and fulfilling experiences, more and more of which will become available to you as you shed off the pounds.

EPILOGUE: WHAT VICTORY TASTES LIKE

I started off this book by quoting Charles Duhigg in The Power of Habit:

*"If you believe you can change - if you make it a
habit - the change becomes real. This is the real
power of habit: The insight that your habits are what
you choose them to be. Once that choice occurs - and
becomes automatic - it's not only real, it starts to
seem inevitable."*

I ended Part One of this book by telling you it will get easier.

Ultimately, the Weight Loss Habit isn't just about changing what you do. It's about changing who you are. Eventually you will become the kind of person who has healthy eating habits.

Here's what's going to happen if you follow the advice I've laid out here: You'll start off slow, or maybe start off quickly with a burst of motivation. As the months go by, you'll pick up more and more healthy habits. And the weight will keep falling away.

Eventually you'll reach your equilibrium weight. You'll be skinny. And you'll keep up your habits that got you there, so you'll stay skinny.

You'll be thrilled by the new you. Amazed at the new energy. You'll probably have more endurance than your friends who have always been skinny, because you're used to hauling around a bunch of extra weight.

But in your mind, you'll still have the self-identity you've built up over a lifetime of being overweight. You'll feel like a fat person in a skinny person's body.

Years will go by. The habits will become automatic. You'll meet people who never knew you before you were skinny, who will be shocked when you tell them you used to be overweight.

And then eventually it will hit you: Your nature has changed. You have changed. You are now a skinny person. Not just externally, but in your soul. And because the decisions that keep you skinny are automatic, you are going to stay skinny for the rest of your life.

The Struggle is gone.

Which brings me to one final autobiographical story.

A few years after I lost the weight, I took a break from work to walk over to Subway and pick up lunch. I ordered my usual six-inch sub, when the sandwich-maker pointed out that because of a special they were having, the footlong would only be fifteen cents more.

My bargain-hunting instincts took over, and since that was obviously a better deal, I agreed to upgrade without really thinking about it. I immediately regretted that decision. I had come in planning on ordering a six-inch sub. Just because it was a good deal wasn't a good reason for me to eat double the calories.

I walked back to the office with my footlong sub, brooding and mad at myself. I knew that I had violated my carefully cultivated habits. Now I had twice as much food as was a good idea.

I was in a foul mood as I sat at my desk to eat. I ate the first half of the sandwich. And then as I looked at the second half, I burst into tears of joy, as I had the realization that I didn't *want* to eat it.

I wasn't making a rational decision that eating it wasn't a good idea. I wasn't exercising willpower. *I simply didn't want it.*

Looking at that half-eaten sandwich was one of the happiest moments of my life. Because that's when I realized all the work I had put in had made me a fundamentally different person. I wasn't a fraud. I wasn't a fat person in a skinny person's body. I wasn't a fool for buying Medium-sized shirts that I'd have to discard as soon as I gained the weight back.

Sitting there at my desk, I knew: I would never be fat again.

DID YOU ENJOY THIS BOOK?

Please rate and review the book on Amazon, and tell a friend about it.

Was there anything you found particularly helpful? Anything you'd like to see added? Anything you didn't like or would want to see changed? I'd love to hear your thoughts. You can reach me at stevenraymarks@gmail.com.

If you like my approach to weight loss, I use a similar approach with self-help in general. You can read my blog at www.selfhelpingyourself.com, and subscribe to my weekly newsletter featuring tips on making self-improvement easier at selfhelpingyourself.com/subscribe.

You can also follow me on Twitter at @YourselfHelping and Instagram at @SelfHelpingYourself.

APPENDIX: FAST FOOD OPTIONS UNDER 600 CALORIES

This section lists meal options that you can find that are under 600 calories at the top 20 fast food restaurants in America, excluding coffee and donut chains. I relied on the nutritional information available on each of the restaurants websites to compile this data. As restaurants often change their offerings and ingredients, actual calorie counts may have changed between when I compiled them and when you read them.

ARBY'S

Note that the sandwiches here are listed without sauce. Arby Sauce adds 15 calories, and Horsey Sauce adds 60 calories.

Most Arby's breakfast items that aren't "Double" or on a "Platter" are under 600 calories.

Item	Calories
Classic Beef 'n Cheddar	450
Classic French Dip and Swiss Au Jus	540
Classic Roast Beef	360
Double Roast Beef	510
Roast Turkey & Swiss Wrap	520
Grand Turkey Club	480
Chopped Farmhouse Salad – Crispy Chicken	430
Chopped Farmhouse Salad – Roast Turkey	240
Salad Dressings	
Light Italian	20
Dijon Honey Mustard	180
Balsamic Vinaigrette	130
Buttermilk Ranch	210

BURGER KING

Item	Calories
Whopper Jr.	310
Quarter Pounder King	580
Hamburger	240
Cheeseburger	280
Double Hamburger	350
Double Cheeseburger	390
Bacon Cheeseburger	320
Bacon Double Cheeseburger	420
Grilled Chicken Sandwich	430
Crispy Chicken Jr	450
Spicy Crispy Chicken Jr	390
Chicken Nuggets	45/nugget
Spicy Chicken Nuggets	55/nugget
Crispy Chicken Tenders	135/piece
Chicken Fries – 9 pc	280

Big Fish Sandwich	510
BK Veggie Burger	390
Garden Chicken Salad Grilled	350+
Club Salad Grilled	450+
Garden Side Salad	60+
Ranch Dressing	260
Italian Dressing	160
Lite Honey Balsamic Vinaigrette	120
Croutons	60
Any CROISSAN'WICH or Biscuit that isn't "Double" or "Fully Loaded"	530 or less

CARL'S JR./HARDEE'S

Note: While Carl's Jr. and Hardee's are the same company, they have some slight differences on their menus. I tried to limit this list to items that were on both menus. In some cases, the nutrition info differed between the two menus, so the numbers that appear before the slash are for Carl's Jr. and after the slash are for Hardee's. Hardee's has many more low-calorie options that were not on the Carl's Jr. menu. If you are interested in reviewing these, you can find them at https://www.hardees.com/nutrition

It is very difficult to find low-calorie breakfast options at Carl's Jr/Hardee's.

Item	Calories
⅓ Pound Lettuce-Wrapped Thickburger	420
Big Hamburger	480
Double Cheeseburger	390
Kid's Hamburger	250
Kid's Cheeseburger	310
Charbroiled Chicken Club Sandwich	590 / 560
Charbroiled BBQ Chicken Sandwich	370 / 350
Spicy Chicken Sandwich	490 / 440
Hand Breaded Chicken Tenders	90/piece

Chicken Stars	45/star
Charbroiled Chicken Salad	280+
Side Salad	140+
House Dressing	210
Blue Cheese Dressing	310
Balsamic Vinaigrette Dressing	20

CHICK-FIL-A

Every one of Chick-Fil-A's sandwiches is under 600 calories, so it's a pretty good option as far as fast food goes. As long as you avoid the sides, drinks, shakes, etc.

Item	Calories
Chicken Sandwich (Spicy / Deluxe / Spicy Deluxe)	440 (450 / 500 / 540)
Nuggets – 8 piece / 12 piece (**Note:** Make sure to add the calories of any dipping sauces to this. Ranch and Chick-Fil-A sauces are 140 calories per cup, and Polynesian is 110 calories. The other sauces are all under 50 calories per cup.)	260 / 390
Chick-n-strips – 3 piece / 4 piece (See note on sauces above)	350 / 470
Grilled Chicken Sandwich (Grilled Chicken Club)	310 (430)
Grilled Nuggets – 8 piece / 12 piece (See note on sauces above)	140 / 210
Grilled Chicken Cool Wrap	350
Grilled Market Salad (no dressing)	330
Cobb Salad (no dressing)	510
Spicy Southwest Salad (no dressing)	450

Salad Dressings	
Light Italian	25
Light Balsamic Vinaigrette	80
Fat Free Honey Mustard	90
Chili Lime Vinaigrette	60
Garlic & Herb Ranch	280
Creamy Salsa	290
Avocado Lime Ranch	310
Apple Cider Vinaigrette	230

All of Chick-Fil-A's breakfast items except for their burritos are under 600 calories.

CHIPOTLE

Since everything is customizable at Chipotle, you have to add up the different ingredients. It is possible to get a reasonably low-calorie meal there, but only if you do a bowl or salad. If you get burritos or tacos, there's just too many calories in the tortillas. And if you get a salad, you have to skip the dressing, which is also high in calories. You can't get guacamole and keep the calories reasonable. Definitely avoid getting chips on the side

Below is a list of how many calories are in each ingredient. I suggest that you sit down and add up the calories from what you like, to come up with something you're satisfied with and is also reasonable calories. Then have this planned ahead of time before you go into the restaurant.

Note that you can ask them for half the usual amount of an ingredient. Though you'll probably end up getting more like two thirds the usual amount, so use two thirds of the calories in your calculation if you're planning to do this.

Item	Calories
Barbacoa	170
Carnitas	210
Chicken	180
Sofritas	150
Steak	150
Rice (Brown or White)	210
Beans (Black or Pinto)	130

Fajita Veggies	20
Tomato Salsa	25
Guacamole	230
Cheese	110
Queso	120
Chili-Corn Salsa	80
Sour Cream	110
Tomatillo Green Chile Salsa	15
Tomatillo Red Chile Salsa	30
Romaine Lettuce	5

DOMINO'S

It's not feasible for me to put together a chart with all the options. But depending on what you get, the hand-tossed pizzas are generally between 250 and 350 calories per slice. Get hand-tossed instead of pan as an easy way to save calories. (Or Brooklyn-style if it's offered in the kind of pizza you're getting.)

If you limit yourself to two slices of a medium hand-tossed pizza, this is reasonably healthy. But seriously ask yourself if it's realistic that you'll be able to cut yourself off after two slices. If not, you should continue to think of pizza as an unhealthy food that you only eat on special occasions.

Alternatively, you could order wings or Specialty Chicken, which are 400–500 calories for a meal.

Be aware that they claim the serving size for their sandwiches and breadbowl pasta is half a sandwich/breadbowl, so these are really double the calories they list on their website. They are not healthy options.

Stay away from the cheesy bread, bread bites, bread twists, and desserts, which are all extremely high in calories.

JACK IN THE BOX

Item	Calories
Hamburger	340
Cheeseburger	380
Jr. Bacon Cheeseburger	480
Jr. Jumbo Jack (with cheese)	420 (460)
Jumbo Jack (with cheese)	520 (600)
Chicken Fajita Pita	350
Chicken Nuggets	50/nugget
Chicken Sandwich (with bacon)	510 (550)
Crispy Chicken Strips	140/piece
Fish Sandwich	410
Jack's Spicy Chicken (with cheese)	550 (630)
Sourdough Grilled Chicken Club	580
Chicken Club Salad – Grilled	370+
Grilled Chicken Salad	250+
Side Salad	20+

Southwest Chicken Salad – grilled with dressing (and corn sticks)	540 (600)
Southwest Dressing	190
Balsamic Vinaigrette Dressing	25
Ranch Dressing	250
Croutons	70
Monster Taco	270
Bacon Ranch Monster Taco	340
Nacho Monster Taco	330
Regular Taco	170
Breakfast Jack (With Bacon) (With Sausage)	350 (380) (500)
Breakfast biscuits	410–550

KFC

The pieces of chicken are generally better than the sandwiches. You can make a huge difference by getting your chicken Kentucky Grilled rather than Original. On the other hand, you'll make a huge difference in the wrong direction if you go Extra Crispy. And be careful with the sides. Biscuits are 180 calories each (before honey or butter), cornbread muffins are 210 calories, potato wedges are 270 calories, and potato salad is 340 calories.

Item	Calories
Chicken Little (Buffalo / Honey BBQ / Nashville Hot)	300 (310 / 320 / 340)
Crispy Colonel Sandwich (Buffalo / Honey BBQ / Nashville Hot)	470 (500 / 510 / 540)
Snack Size Famous Bowl	270
Original Chicken Breast (Extra Crispy / Spicy Crispy / Kentucky Grilled)	390 (530 / 350 / 210)
Original Chicken Drumstick (Extra Crispy / Spicy Crispy / Kentucky Grilled)	130 (170 / 130 / 80)
Original Chicken Thigh (Extra Crispy / Spicy Crispy / Kentucky Grilled)	280 (330 / 270 / 150)
Original Chicken Whole Wing (Extra Crispy / Spicy Crispy / Kentucky Grilled)	130 (170 / 120 / 70)
Corn on the Cob	70

| Green Beans | 25 |
| Sweet Kernel Corn | 70 |

MCDONALD'S

Item	Calories
Hamburger	250
Cheeseburger	300
Double Cheeseburger	440
McDouble	390
Quarter Pounder With Cheese	510
Big Mac	540
Filet-O-Fish	390
McChicken	400
McRib	500
Artisan Grilled Chicken Sandwich	430
Chicken McNuggets	45/nugget
Buttermilk Crispy Tenders	120/piece
Bacon Ranch Grilled Chicken Salad with ranch dressing	440
Southwest Grilled Chicken Salad with dressing	440
Side Salad	15+

Ranch Dressing (Remember you can use part of this to reduce the calories – ½ the packet would be ½ the calories.)	140
Southwest Dressing	110
Vinaigrette Dressing	40
Fruit N Yogurt Parfait	210
Egg McMuffin	300
All other breakfast sandwiches	420–550

PANDA EXPRESS

Typically at Panda Express, people get a Bowl, which comes with either fried rice or chow mein, or a Plate which comes with a serving of each. (Or two servings of one of these.) It's not going to be possible to get a reasonable portion of food if you do this. The chow mein is 510 calories, and the fried rice is 520. If you get the Plate, you're already over 1,000 calories before you've even ordered your main dishes.

However, instead of getting the chow mein and fried rice, you can get their Super Greens, which are only 90 calories per serving. If you do that, it's possible to eat a reasonably healthy meal at Panda Express. Otherwise, the only way to do it is to split your take-home Bowl or Plate into multiple meals.

In general, it's better to stay away from anything that is fried or breaded. This includes a lot of their signature dishes, such as Orange Chicken, Beijing Beef, and Honey Sesame Chicken.

Every item on Panda's menu is under 600 calories, but since you'll likely be eating multiple items, I'm only going to list those that are less than 300 calories.

Item	Calories
Black Pepper Chicken	280
Kung Pao Chicken	290
Mushroom Chicken	220
Potato Chicken	190
String Bean Chicken	190

Broccoli Beef	150
Firecracker Shrimp	110
Chicken Egg Roll	200
Grilled Teriyaki Chicken	300
Grilled Asian Chicken	300
Sweet and Sour Chicken	300

PANERA BREAD

Despite having a somewhat healthy image, Panera tends to serve large amounts of food, or food that contains a lot of high-calorie bread. It's hard to find lower calorie options. They do offer half-sandwiches, but realistically you're not going to eat that. Even most of their salads are over 600 calories once you add dressing. And you definitely want to avoid their bread bowls, or sides of bread.

On the other hand, almost all of their breakfast options are under 600 calories. Because they have such an extensive menu, I'm not going to list them all.

If you do find yourself at Panera Bread for lunch or dinner, here are the few low-calorie options I could find.

Item	Calories
Mediterranean Grain Bowl (No meat)	590
Mediterranean Veggie on Tomato Basil	470
Steak and Arugula on Sourdough	480
Turkey on Whole Grain	540
Asian Sesame Salad with Chicken (With Dressing)	410 (500)
Caesar Salad (With Dressing / With Chicken and Dressing)	320 (490 / 620)
Seasonal Greens Salad – No Dressing (This is low enough calorie that you can add the dressing of your choice and still keep it under 600 calories.)	190
Spicy Thai Salad With Chicken (With Dressing)	460 (510)

PIZZA HUT

Pizza Hut is very similar to Dominos. However, they have personal pan pizzas, which make it a bit easier to get reasonable portions. The Cheese, Hawaiian, Pepperoni (not Pepperoni Lover's), and Veggie Lover's are all 600 calories or under. And most of the other personal pan pizzas aren't too much over 600 calories. They range from 640 for the Buffalo Chicken to 840 for the Meat Lover's.

Avoid their pastas, p'zones, and sandwiches, which have enormous amounts of calories. Even their "Smaller Appetites" menu is high-calorie.

Some of their salads are lower calorie (though some aren't), but who orders salads from Pizza Hut?

Wings are 80–100 calories per wing depending on options, unless you get the Smoky Garlic wings which are 110–120 calories, or the Garlic Parmesan which are 130–140 calories.

POPEYE'S

There are lots of options here if you avoid the sides, or stick with green beans as your side. Also, this is a good example of coleslaw having way more calories than you would expect. (As discussed in the chapter on high calorie "healthy" foods.) Popeye's coleslaw has more calories than their macaroni and cheese, and twice as much as their mashed potatoes.

Also, be careful about their dipping sauces, as most are in the 100–150 calorie range. The Barbecue sauce is okay at 45 calories, and the cocktail sauce is okay at 30 calories.

Item	Calories
Wing – Mild or Spicy	210
Leg – Mild / Spicy	160 / 170
Thigh – Mild / Spicy	280 / 260
Breast – Mild / Spicy	440 / 420
Nuggets – 4 pc / 6 pc	150 / 230
Tenders – Mild / Spicy / Naked	340 / 310 / 170
Spicy Chicken Sandwich	480
Chicken Wrap – Loaded / Naked	310 / 200
Naked BBQ Chicken Po' Boy	340
Popcorn Shrimp	330

Butterfly Shrimp – 8 pc	290
Catfish Fillet	460

SONIC

The Nutritional information Sonic puts out tries to bewilder you with options, by giving separate listings for if you get your burger with ketchup, or mustard, or mayo, or ketchup and mayo, etc. To simplify this, a good rule of thumb is that adding mayo adds about 100 calories. The difference between ketchup and mustard is negligible. Assume any item on this chart has ketchup if that's an option, and does not have mayo.

Stay away from their blasts and shakes, some of which can top 1,500 (!) calories. Also their Cherry Limeades are shockingly high in calories, unless you get the diet version.

Item	Calories
Sonic Burger	540
Sonic Cheeseburger	600
Hatch Green Chile Cheeseburger	590
Jr. Burger	330
Quarter Pound Double Cheeseburger (I don't know why the Quarter Pound Double Cheeseburger is fewer calories than the regular cheeseburger. My guess would be less fixings or a smaller bun. Anyway, here's a way you can feel like you're eating more while consuming fewer calories.)	570
Veggie Burger	440
BLT Toaster Sandwich	580

Chicken Wrap Grilled (Crispy)	480 (570)
6 pc. Boneless Wings – Buffalo (Honey BBQ) (Sweet Asian Chile)	440 (470) (470)
Classic Chicken Sandwich – Grilled (Crispy)	470 (550)
Crispy Tender Sandwich	440
Jumbo Popcorn Chicken – Small (Medium)	330 (490)
Crispy Tenders – 3 pc. (5 pc.)	260 (430)
Fish Sandwich	540
Grilled Cheese Sandwich	430
6" Hot Dogs	320–470, depending on options
Breakfast Burrito – Ham / Bacon / Sausage	440 / 470 / 500
Brioche Breakfast Sandwich – Ham / Bacon	470 / 530
Croissonic Breakfast Sandwich – Ham / Bacon	490 / 560

SUBWAY

As of the time I'm writing this, every six-inch sub on Subway's menu that doesn't include guacamole or the word "Ultimate" in its name is under 600 calories. Rather than copying Subway's entire menu, I'll just tell you to avoid those few items, and stick to the six-inch subs instead of the footlongs. The footlong subs are double the calories of the six-inch subs, obviously.

Also, skip the cookies, which are over 200 calories each, and they sell them in packs of three. Which means there's more calories in your dessert than in the entire rest of your meal.

You can find more information on how many calories are in each specific item on Subway's menu here: https://www.subway.com/en-US/MenuNutrition/Nutrition/NutritionGrid

TACO BELL

Taco Bell has plenty of lower calorie items. Unfortunately, people often get multiple items. To stay under 600 calories, you'll have to limit yourself to one mid-sized item, a small burrito plus a taco, or three tacos. Or you could replace a taco with Cinnabon delights, which in my personal opinion is the best dessert at any fast food place.

Item	Calories
7-layer burrito	420
Bean Burrito	350
Beefy 5-Layer Burrito	490
Beefy Fritos Burrito	440
Beefy Nacho Loaded Griller	370
Burrito Supreme	390
Cheese Bean & Rice Burrito	410
Cheese Potato Griller	340
Shredded Chicken Burrito	420
Cheesy Roll Up	180
Shredded Chicken Quesadilla Melt	310
Spicy Tostada	190

Power Menu Bowl – Veggie / Chicken / Steak	430 / 480 / 490
Chalupa Supreme	350
Cheesy Gordita Crunch	500
Crunchwrap Supreme	530
Gordita Supreme	280
Mexican Pizza	530
Meximelt	250
Nachos Supreme	430
Quesadilla (with chicken or steak)	450 (500)
Crunchy Taco (Supreme)	170 (190)
Soft Taco (Supreme)	180 (210)
Spicy Potato Soft Taco	230
Doritos Locos Taco (Supreme)	170 (190)
Cinnabon Delights (2-pack)	160

WENDY'S

Item	Calories
Dave's Single	570
Jr. Bacon Cheeseburger	380
Double Stack	390
Jr. Hamburger (Cheeseburger / Cheeseburger Deluxe)	240 (280 / 340)
Grilled Bacon Jalapeno Chicken Sandwich	600
Chicken Nuggets – 4pc / 6pc / 10 pc (Spicy 4 pc / 6 pc / 10 pc)	170 / 250 / 420 (190 / 280 / 470)
Grilled Barbecue Chicken Sandwich	520
Grilled Avocado BLT Chicken Sandwich	600
Homestyle Chicken Sandwich / Spicy Chicken Sandwich	500
Grilled Chicken Sandwich (Crispy Chicken Sandwich) *This is a rare case where the crispy version has fewer calories than the grilled version, because it is smaller*	370 (330)
Grilled Asiago Ranch Club	520

Crispy Chicken BLT	420
Chicken Wrap – Grilled / Crispy	300 / 370
Spicy Buffalo Chicken Salad – Half Size	430
Parmesan Chicken Salad – Half / Full	310 / 560
Southwest Avocado Chicken Salad – Half / Full	300 / 600
Taco Salad – Half / Full	430 / 610
Apple Pecan Chicken Salad – Half / Full	340 / 570
Egg and Swiss Croissant – Bacon / Sausage	430 / 600
Maple Bacon Chicken Croissant	570
Egg and Cheese Biscuit – Bacon / Sausage	450 / 630
Sausage Biscuit	500
Honey Butter Chicken Biscuit	510
Classic Egg and Cheese Sandwich – Bacon / Sausage	330 / 500

130

ABOUT THE AUTHOR

Steven Ray Marks started his childhood wealthy, then suddenly switched to being raised by a poor single mother working nights after his attorney father got caught stealing from his clients. He has a BA in Economics from Georgetown University, and an MFA in Screenwriting from The University of Southern California. He switches between writing and accounting. He has been the Controller for several startups, and wrote video games based on Hannah Montana, High School Musical, and Are You Smarter Than A Fifth Grader.

He grew up obese, then in his mid-20s figured out an effective strategy for losing weight, and has kept the weight off since. He currently lives in Los Angeles with his wife and an ever-changing number of foster kittens.

He blogs about making self-improvement easier at SelfHelpingYourself.com.

Info
Books and writing projects: www.stevenraymarks.com
Self-Improvement Blog: www.selfhelpingyourself.com
Twitter: @YourselfHelping
Instagram: @SelfHelpingYourself
E-mail: stevenraymarks@gmail.com

www.ingramcontent.com/pod-product-compliance
Lightning Source LLC
Chambersburg PA
CBHW051456250726
48655CB00001B/449